D0656569

BUILD YOUR OWN BODY

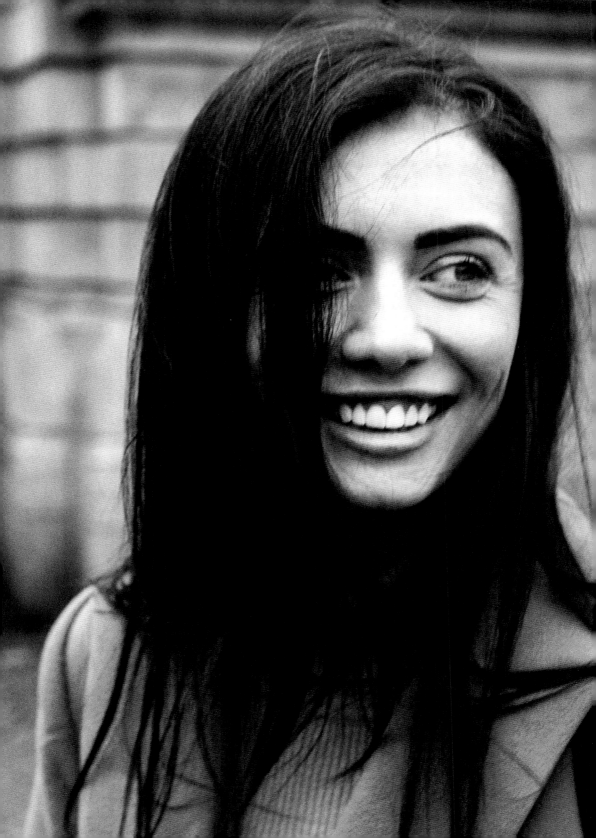

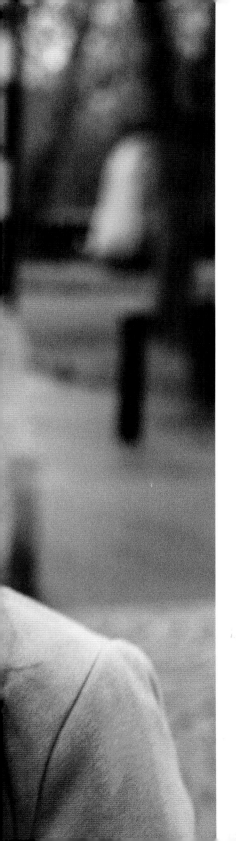

THE AUTHOR

Kelly Donegan is an online fitness influencer and competitive bodybuilder with a passion for weightlifting and physical challenges. The Tallaght native found public notoriety in 2011 after appearing on Ireland's most controversial reality TV show. Finding herself unhappy with life's pressures and stereotypes, Kelly turned to fitness – and never looked back. Little did she know that fitness would become her passion, saviour and a source of empowerment.

JOIN KELLY ONLINE:

#BYOB

#BUILDYOUROWNBODY

FACEBOOK: KELLY DONEGAN

INSTAGRAM: ITSKELLYDONEGAN

TWITTER: ITSKELLYDONEGAN

YOUTUBE: KELLY DONEGAN

WEBSITE: WWW.KELLYDONEGAN.IE

Gill Books
Hume Avenue
Park West
Dublin 12
www.gillbooks.ie

Gill Books is an imprint of M.H. Gill and Co.

© Kelly Donegan 2016

978 07171 7031 9

Edited by Kristin Jensen and Ruth Mahony
Designed by AmpVisual.com
Photography by Gavin Glave
Cover shoot styled by Courtney Smith
Cover shoot make-up by Sineád Murphy
Cover shoot hair styling by Alison O'Leary
Shot on location at Chocolate Factory,
26 King's Inn Street, Dublin 1 and
FLYEfit, 63 South Great George's Street, Dublin 2
Printed by BZ Graf. S.A., Poland

This book is typeset in Avenir Next Condensed.

The paper used in this book comes from the wood pulp of managed forests.
For every tree felled, at least one tree is planted, thereby renewing natural resources.

All rights reserved.
No part of this publication may be copied, reproduced or transmitted in any form or by
any means, without written permission of the publishers.

A CIP catalogue record for this book is available from the British Library.

5 4 3 2 1

Note from the Publisher
This book is written as a source of information only and is not intended to be taken as
a replacement for medical advice. A qualified medical practitioner should always be
consulted before beginning any new diet, exercise or health plan.

BUILD YOUR OWN BODY

STRONG IS THE NEW SKINNY
KELLY DONEGAN

Gill Books

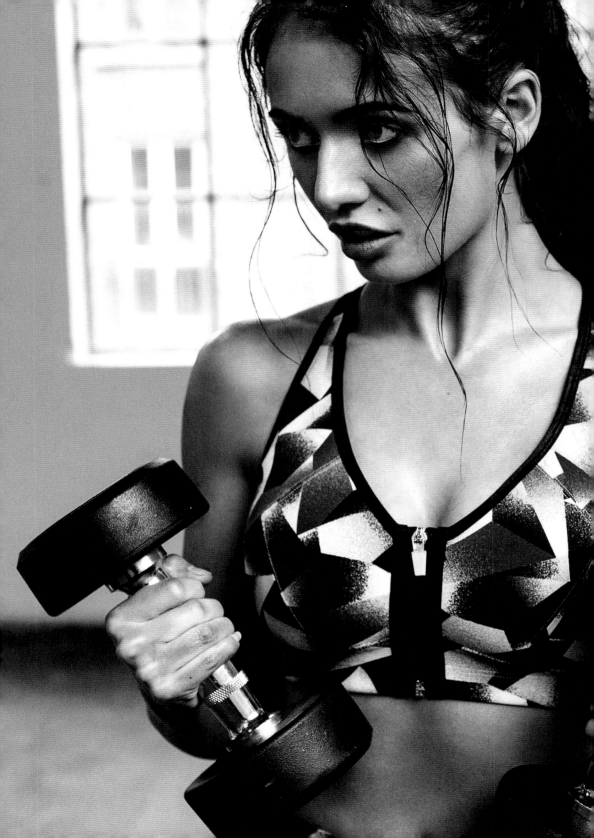

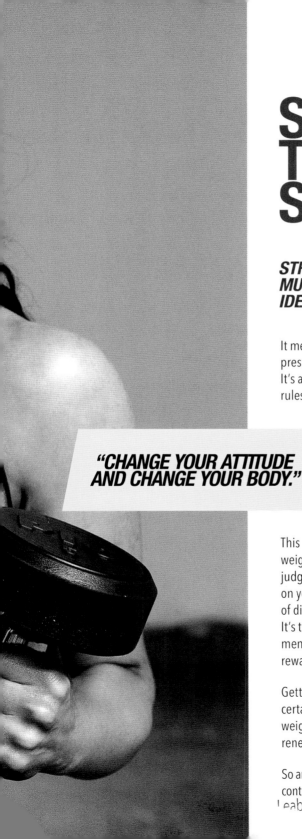

STRONG IS THE NEW SKINNY

STRONG IS THE NEW SKINNY IS SO MUCH MORE THAN A PHRASE OR AN IDEA. IT'S A REVOLUTION.

It means throwing away all the old stereotypes and pressures around what the female body should look like. It's about building a body that *you* want. You make the rules and you set the standards.

> **"CHANGE YOUR ATTITUDE AND CHANGE YOUR BODY."**

It's time to stop idealising an unrealistic body image and to stop comparing your physical beauty to other women. Size zero, thigh gaps, a skin-and-bones physique and weakness are out. Strong, powerful, hardworking and healthy are in.

This revolution means embracing the power of weightlifting and exercise. In this world you won't be judged on your looks or your body, but you will be judged on your efforts and your ability to persevere in the face of difficulty. Strong isn't a luxury just for men any more. It's time for women to be strong too, both physically and mentally, to get healthy and to kick ass in the gym. The rewards will be an improved body and mind.

Getting strong doesn't mean getting bulky, and it certainly doesn't mean becoming masculine. The modern weightlifting woman looks sexier than ever and has a renewed self-confidence.

So are you ready to join the strong revolution and take back control of your life, your mind and your body?

Leabharlanna Poiblí Chathair Bhaile Átha Cliath
Dublin City Public Libraries

ACKNOWLEDGEMENTS

Most books tend to end with thank yous, but for me this book has to start with them because I wouldn't be the person I am without all of these people and I certainly wouldn't be writing this inspirational book.

Firstly, thank you to Gill Books for believing in me and for giving me a new platform to share my knowledge and my story. It's probably the most exciting and meaningful yes of my career and has reaffirmed my belief in never giving up. For those who think the big yes will never come, don't quit because the right one will work out for you, usually when you least expect it. Thanks to the wonderful team at Gill Books I worked with on *Build Your Own Body*. They supported me from day one and made the experience so unbelievably special. Thank you to Nicki, Ruth, Kristin, Emma and Teresa.

To my mam, Susan, who I know deep down has always been my biggest fan, thank you for supporting me and keeping me grounded. I can't imagine it's easy having a daughter like me, who seems to pick the most unusual and risky routes in life, so for being the most wonderful, caring, selfless, patient woman on the planet, thank you. Thank you to my dad, John, who inspires me to work hard on a daily basis and who reminds me to never forget to just be silly and to laugh no matter what age you are. Thank you both for being amazing parents. I wouldn't be the person I am today without your love, support and craziness.

To my sister Mollie and my brother Craig, who bring laughter and madness into my life, who don't take any rubbish from me and always find new and creative ways to annoy me. I am so lucky that I can call my brother and sister best friends, so thank you.

To my best friend, Grace, there aren't enough pages in this book to fit all the reasons why I need to thank you. You have been my rock, my shoulder to cry on and my solace in my saddest days. I am forever grateful for your friendship, your love and your kindness. I am truly blessed that I get to call you my best friend.

To my coach, Calin, thank you for helping me discover my inner athlete, for pushing me to be my best and for being my teacher.

To all of my family and friends, thank you for everything. I am fortunate to have so many wonderful people in my life who have been there for me.

To my dog, Tyson, who kept me company every day while I was writing this book and for proving that sometimes all a girl needs is her dog.

This may seem a little strange (but hey, my book was always going to be somewhat abnormal), but I want to say a big thank you to the universe for all of the tough times, the sad days, the dark days, the times I wanted to quit, the times that tested me, the past people in my life and for all the nos I've received over the years. Positive life situations are important and exciting, but it's the negative times that build character, that push you to dig deep and to keep fighting. I have discovered just how strong I am as a result of all of these things and they are an important part of my journey. They say that life deals you the cards that it thinks you can handle and that the hard times allow you to discover your inner warrior, so I have to be grateful and acknowledge them. My past has made me who I am today.

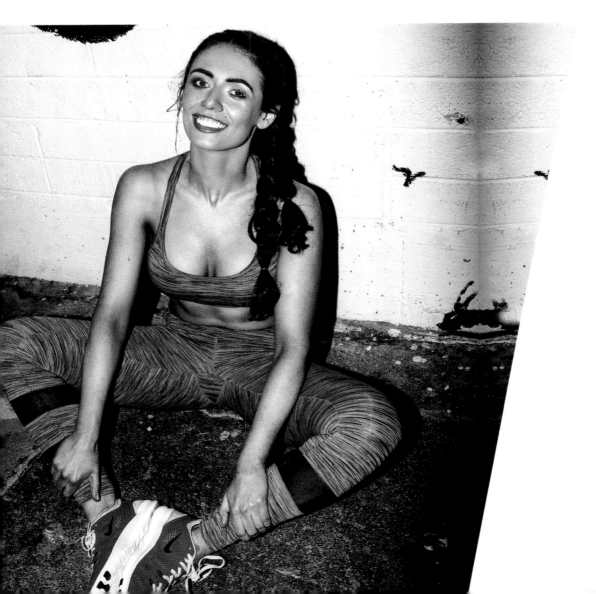

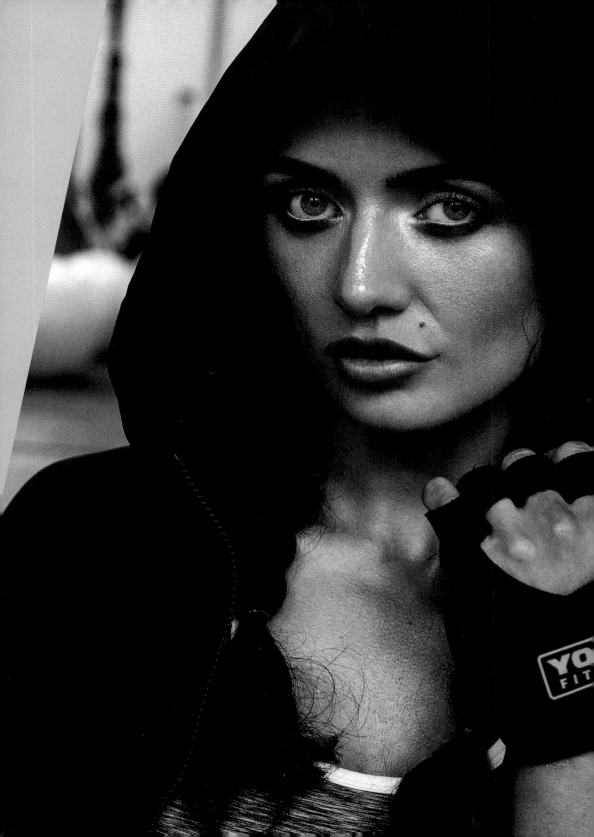

CONTENTS

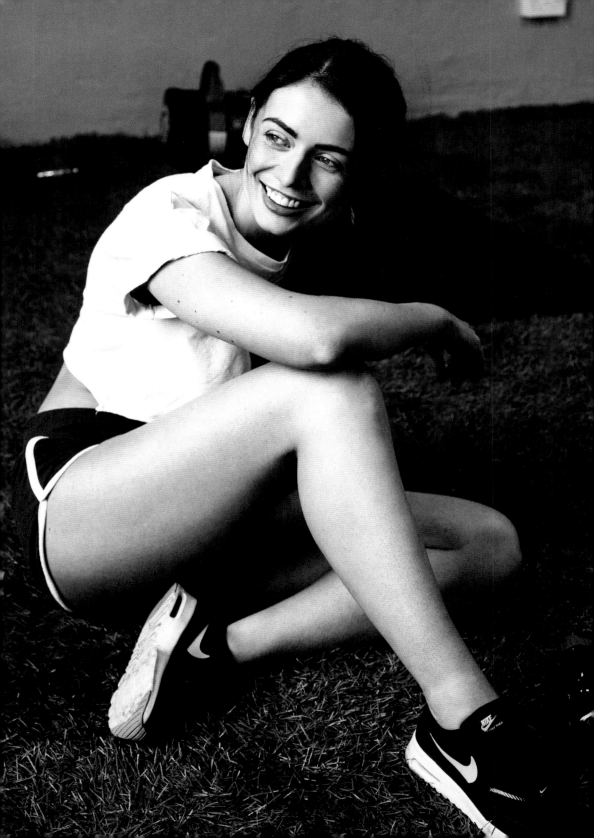

FOREWORD

I have over two decades of experience working in the world of fitness and bodybuilding. My career started in my home country of Romania, where I studied sports management and physical education before becoming a PE teacher. My passion for bodybuilding started many years ago, before making Ireland my home.

I have trained many clients and athletes over the years and pride myself on helping them through my own experience and knowledge. Five years ago I launched my own nutrition company and created Team Titan Ireland, a group of select men and women who compete at national and international level in a range of bodybuilding categories under my supervision and guidance. Kelly is a part of this team, but before that she was a friend, one who has gone on to become one of the most important athletes on our team.

Kelly always makes it her business to support her fellow teammates. She constantly inspires and motivates others and is a dream athlete to work with.

She is the epitome of hard work and dedication. She sticks to every challenge that she faces as a competitive bodybuilder, whether it's diet or training. She is always trying to learn new ways to improve or push herself and to take her body to the next level.

There are no airs or graces to this girl, just hard work and focus. She has totally embraced the world of fitness and bodybuilding since we started in 2013. Her ambition to inspire others continues to impress me, and her sharp mind for business and her creativity will see this lady gain huge success. She has a bright future ahead of her in the world of fitness and I am looking forward to watching her journey.

I recommend this book to anyone looking to be inspired and who wants to get fit. Kelly has made it happen for herself time and time again – she has transformed her own body from skinny to strong. She knows what she is talking about because she puts it into practice every day.

– Calin Brehaita, owner of Titan Nutrition Ireland and International Federation of Bodybuilding and Fitness (IFBB) professional judge.

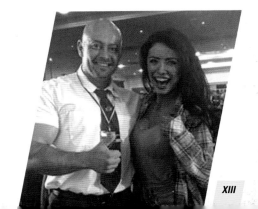

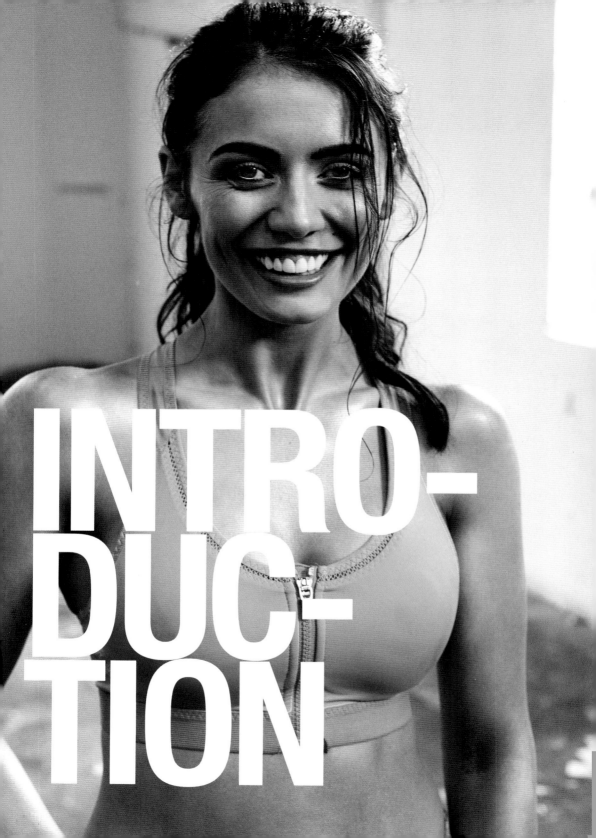

INTRO-DUC-TION

BYOB simply means build your own body, because the reality is that building your own body is simple – that is, of course, with the right information, plan, support and determination.

This book will help you get started. It will hopefully clear up the confusion surrounding getting fit, losing weight, lifting weights and putting on muscle. It will share some important theory and also give you useful tips to stay on track and help you build the body of your dreams, whatever that may be. Whether you want to drop a couple pounds ahead of your holidays or make long-term changes, this book will help you understand how to do it. It will teach you the language of fitness, give you the confidence to follow through with your goals and help you to understand *why* you are doing things rather than just telling you to do it. It will cover some basics of nutrition and supplements, exercise techniques, diet plans and everything in between. **My hope is that after you've read this book, you'll not only have confidence in yourself, but that you'll also have confidence in fitness and in what it can do for you.**

I also want you to use fitness as a tool for happiness and empowerment. It will help you say goodbye to the standards set by society. I want you to be strong, feel strong and radiate strong. This book will give you the information, the support and the motivation you need to get started, but you are going to have to do the work to take back control of your fitness regime and earn the body you have always wanted. *BYOB* is a book for strong women who want to train hard, get their hands dirty and who aren't afraid to work up a sweat.

Over the last two years, I have learned so much about fitness and nutrition and now I want to help you to see just how easy and fun getting fit can be. During that time I have received endless emails, private messages and Instagram comments asking me my secrets and tips, but the truth is that there are no secrets to getting fit. It's just hard work and dedication along with honest information, which is what I'm going to share with you here.

There is no limit to the amount of information you can learn about the body and how it works, how food reacts with your system and how exercise impacts on your health. I'm still learning as I go along, but I take a huge amount of pride in what I do know because I have put it into practice. I know how to get in shape because I've done it – and it has changed my life.

This isn't a bikini bodybuilding manual, but it does incorporate some of the things I've learned from being a competitive bodybuilder, like the importance of having good information, a good plan and a good mental attitude. Being super fit isn't just for fitness experts, athletes and professionals, and you don't need to spend thousands on a dietician to understand how to have a healthy, balanced diet. Your results are 100% down to you. There is only so much a coach, a personal trainer or a nutritionist can do for you. *You* **have to make it happen.**

Are you ready?

"DON'T WISH FOR YOUR DREAM BODY — WORK FOR IT."

MY STORY

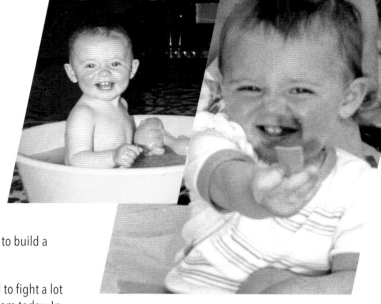

I'm pinching myself to think that I can now call myself an author, a fitness motivator, a competitive bodybuilder who has represented her country, an online influencer with thousands of followers and a self-confident woman on a mission to build a fitness empire, one goal at a time.

But it wasn't always this way. I've had to fight a lot of demons to be the Kelly Donegan I am today. In fact, writing this book has made me answer a lot of questions about myself and helped me come to terms with the hard times and the obstacles I have faced. I hope my honesty and my journey will resonate with you and that it will inspire you too to get fit and healthy.

If you follow me online, you may have already taken this journey with me. You might see me as the reality TV personality turned fitness badass, but there are so many more layers to my story and it goes much further back in time. I don't even think my closest friends know just how low I was or how I feel about my past, because I've always been a pretty positive person who just sucks it up and gets on with things. My new calling in the world of fitness is only a result of hitting rock bottom and having to totally change my mindset. *BYOB* is a positive book about building the body of your dreams,

about how amazing fitness can be and about the power of being healthy, but before I had the option to help you build your own body, I had to build myself back up from scratch.

> **"SOMETIMES YOU HAVE TO HIT ROCK BOTTOM TO DISCOVER YOUR TRUE INNER STRENGTH."**

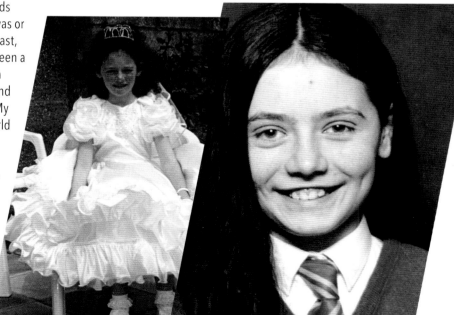

LET'S START AT THE BEGINNING

Let's go back to the very beginning, to Kelly the diehard tomboy who loved being outside and playing football on my cul-de-sac with my neighbours, who had a flair for drawing and painting and who, bizarrely, collected rubber animals, from horses to tigers.

But as a young child I was also very quiet and had huge issues speaking in front of people. Anyone who knows me now will laugh at that, because today I love nothing more than speaking to a packed room and inspiring people. I struggled so much as a child that I had to attend special English classes with the foreign national students to help me build my confidence and improve my speaking skills.

Growing up, I was never the typical girly girl. Even as I got older, I preferred my Nintendo over the Tamagotchi, where I was master of games such as Super Mario World and Super Ghouls 'n' Ghosts (there's some major nostalgia there for you, folks). I was also an enthusiastic Pokémon fan and I loved a Japanese anime show, *Sailor Moon*, and the Spice Girls – the only two things that reminded me that I was, in fact, a girl.

The only major difference between me and any other young adult about to make the transition to the early teenage years was that I suffered from eczema and asthma. Being a wheezy, flaky, red and scaly child really wasn't too much of an issue, even though there were days I couldn't breathe or run fast enough and times when my skin was itchy and raw, but I was too busy pretending I was a horse to give a damn that I was different.

But between the ages of eight and 12, I became more aware of who was popular, who was pretty, who had nice things and who had interesting stories. I realised that there was nothing that special about me, except for being the girl who had a big horrible rash all over her face and body. It's weird when you become aware of body image and feel the pressure even at such a young age. It sucks, actually. Obviously, what I thought about myself wasn't true. Of course I was interesting; I just didn't feel that way in comparison to the other girls in my class and year.

My feelings of inadequacy continued into secondary school, where the pressures of young womanhood become even more apparent. I was this dorky girl with dry, horrible skin everywhere, I didn't have the latest clothes and I didn't go to a hairdresser once a month for a half head of highlights like the rest of the popular girls did.

I still remember the first day of secondary school, when we were asked what we would like to be when we got older. I wrote down a vet, an artist or a model. At that time in my life I felt like I was an invisible, unimportant and utterly uninteresting nobody. But in my mind, a model was beautiful, popular and had this exciting, wonderful life – the exact opposite of me. I know this all sounds daft, but hey, I was 12 and silly, and that was my mindset. I wish I could take a time machine back to that girl and tell her to snap out of it and to realise that she *was* important, that she was hilarious and a talented young artist.

Unfortunately, my years of feeling invisible led me down the path that every parent hopes their teen bypasses (sorry, Mum and Dad!). Being popular and having a great social life became my priorities and the rest of my life suffered. I quickly made many friends. Every day was exciting, usually because I was in some kind of trouble. But even after my transition from dorky, boyish nobody to freedom-loving rebel, underneath it all I still felt like a fraud because deep down I knew I was just a fake. I wasn't popular, I wasn't cool. I was still the insecure girl covered in eczema.

I look back and wonder why I made life so complicated for myself. I probably caused many of my skin breakouts just from my own actions. The only thing that stopped me from plunging into total failure as a teenager was my commitment to extracurricular activities, which helped me look like I was still a normal member of society and a somewhat upstanding citizen and student. Since childhood I have dabbled in a colourful array of hobbies and interests, art being the only consistent one. I went from ballroom dancing to horse-riding enthusiast, tin whistle player extraordinaire and member of the secondary school trad band, right wing for the school hockey team and proud member of the school choir, singing as an alto (which means you actually sing like a man). I even managed to discover my inner leader as debs organiser. At least I can say I did something positive with my teenage years.

As a teenager, I was taller than most of the girls in my year and sported a size six body, but I had overwhelming insecurities: I had no curves, I had the flattest bum in existence and I had a minus A bra size. I could never just be content with what I had. I remember trying to go on a diet once that consisted of Cookie Crisp cereal, joining aerobics and also trying the starvation diet, which lasted about six hours. I wish someone had helped me understand myself a little better and had taught me about the importance of good food and exercise. Daily exercise and a healthy diet may have helped with the difficulties of being a teenager.

I survived school and the Leaving Certificate and somehow managed to get myself to art college. Art has always been one of my biggest passions and it was the only class I can say I was a straight A student in, so it seemed like the logical choice for college and the only option for my future. But I had no idea what I wanted from the world or what I wanted my career to be. I was still that same insecure girl who felt invisible. I still had the small dream of *actually* being somebody important and doing something unique, but I was still lost.

I found it very difficult to apply myself in college, and like most students I enjoyed the party scene a little too much. I may have been lost, but boy did I enjoy living the creative life of an art student addicted to techno music and wild parties. I was doing the typical student thing: college, partying and working two jobs, retail slave midweek and promo girl every weekend. I actually don't know how I balanced so many things at once. But all the distraction of fun and mischief allowed me to become more confident and I even signed up for a beauty pageant. The original dorky kid in a beauty pageant – who would have ever imagined?

THE REALITY TV YEARS

It felt unreal, considering my long-held dream of getting into modelling and proving to myself that I was in fact important. I was optimistic that they wouldn't realise I was a total fraud and certainly not a quintessential beauty. Even though the pageant totally went against my true nature as a sports-loving tomboy, I got a lot out of the experience. My self-confidence was at an all-time high, and for the first time, life seemed pretty decent. I worked in some exciting modelling jobs, I got to be the glamorous girl and to the outside world my life seemed unbelievable. I even managed to find myself on a TV show watched by hundreds of thousands of Irish people.

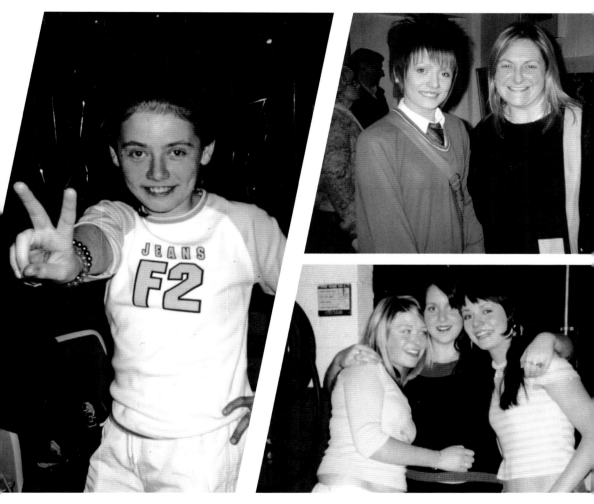

Of course, when you get into this type of industry, the pressures include how slim you are, whether or not you have a thigh gap and a naturally big chest and how many followers you have on Twitter or Instagram – total toxic malarkey that can shatter your perception of what's real and important. Oh, and don't worry – my original low body confidence is still lurking in the shadows and I'm still the proud owner of a crusty skin condition.

For the first time I discovered what it's like to be publicly criticised, but it was no skin off my nose because I was my own worst critic anyway. I have

got remarks online discussing how big my nose is, how my teeth look like a bomb has gone off in my mouth and how my head looks like a melted welly boot. I think these kinds of statements are hysterical now, but back then they were a real punch in the gut.

People ask me all the time what it was like to be on a TV show. It was a totally surreal experience, filled with excitement and drama. By no means did I think I was a celebrity, but it did seem like everybody in Ireland knew who I was overnight. It all happened very fast and all anybody could talk about was this new TV show. It was very exciting to be a part of it. I felt like things in my life were going to get really exciting, both financially and personally.

Unfortunately, that wasn't the case. Yes, I got a lot of publicity, but I wasn't excited about the person that people saw. I also found myself with fewer opportunities than ever before. I was on a rollercoaster ride of ups and downs. I had lost a huge part of myself: that sporty, down-to-earth, funny, relaxed girl who I hadn't appreciated in the past. I no longer had any hobbies or outlets to just vent. If only I'd had fitness back then.

In theory I got exactly what I wanted, but it didn't translate into success, happiness or a comfortable life. Life was a mess. All my years of trying to be somebody else finally caught up with me and I was miserable. I found myself in a dark hole that only seemed to get deeper any time I tried to climb out of it. There was a period of time when I felt like I would wake up in the morning, open my eyes in bed, then I would blink and I was back in bed again, going to sleep.

I felt hopeless. I felt like a failure. I was shattered, both mentally and physically. I didn't even care if I was alive. I saw people my age going off on holidays, with reliable careers and in happy relationships, but I had nothing. Every now and then I managed to drag myself out of the house, usually only to walk my dog with the odd flutter to an event or to see a friend. This was always a bad idea, because I'd have to pretend I was okay, that life was super. Yet again I was a fraud with a smile on my face and a pocketful of meaningless words to share with people who asked how I was or what I was up to.

I felt like life was beating me so hard that I didn't have the energy to fight back. Every time I tried to take a step forward, I would get knocked back even harder. I felt hard done by and couldn't comprehend why life was so difficult and challenging. It almost felt like the world had taken some personal vendetta out against me.

I eventually decided to let go of any aspect of my life that was negative or in any way toxic. That included anything that didn't represent me in a good light, because the truth was that I was just a chilled out, artistic soul that needed balance. Being a glamour girl just wasn't me.

All the years of being unhappy with myself caught up with me and I had to face it head on. It took a long time for me to realise that I had to do something, even though I was still depressed, low and lacking in confidence. I think the only thing that kept me from totally plummeting into suicidal thoughts was my weekly charity work with Dogs Aid Animal Rescue. It's something I'm so grateful for and I genuinely encourage anyone who is struggling to do something for somebody else – in my case, it was fundraising for animals in need.

I also met some amazing people who offered me laughs and support at a time when I struggled to crack a smile. Just by doing something, things started to change a little and I found myself wanting to explore new avenues. Sure, I had all the time in the world because my life was fairly empty.

THE TURNING POINT

I decided I was going to start a fitness blog as an outlet for me to express myself and explore a new avenue. Before hitting my low point, I had found fitness quite interesting. As a tomboy at heart, it had always called to me. I knew very little

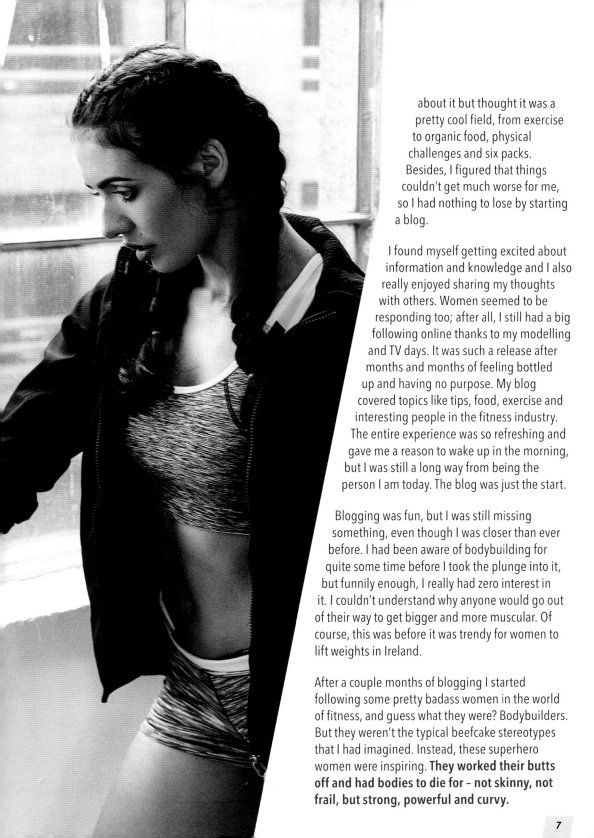

about it but thought it was a pretty cool field, from exercise to organic food, physical challenges and six packs. Besides, I figured that things couldn't get much worse for me, so I had nothing to lose by starting a blog.

I found myself getting excited about information and knowledge and I also really enjoyed sharing my thoughts with others. Women seemed to be responding too; after all, I still had a big following online thanks to my modelling and TV days. It was such a release after months and months of feeling bottled up and having no purpose. My blog covered topics like tips, food, exercise and interesting people in the fitness industry. The entire experience was so refreshing and gave me a reason to wake up in the morning, but I was still a long way from being the person I am today. The blog was just the start.

Blogging was fun, but I was still missing something, even though I was closer than ever before. I had been aware of bodybuilding for quite some time before I took the plunge into it, but funnily enough, I really had zero interest in it. I couldn't understand why anyone would go out of their way to get bigger and more muscular. Of course, this was before it was trendy for women to lift weights in Ireland.

After a couple months of blogging I started following some pretty badass women in the world of fitness, and guess what they were? Bodybuilders. But they weren't the typical beefcake stereotypes that I had imagined. Instead, these superhero women were inspiring. **They worked their butts off and had bodies to die for – not skinny, not frail, but strong, powerful and curvy.**

I became totally obsessed with these athletes who defied all the stereotypes of what women should look like. In complete contrast to the typical media personalities on the covers of glossy magazines who made me look at my body and hate it, these women motivated me. Now, instead of seeing a celebrity on the cover of a magazine and presuming she had a dietician and a personal trainer or comparing myself to the girl who seems to be naturally gifted with a body from the gods, I was looking at women who were getting to the gym at 5am before work or college, preparing all their own food and working out like machines as well as balancing their everyday life. To me, this seemed so much more real and achievable. If these normal women were kicking ass, then why couldn't I?

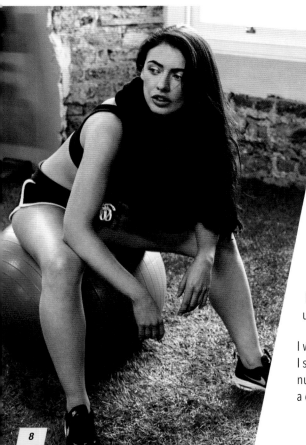

I decided to enter my first bodybuilding competition around November 2013 and was fortunate to already have access to a bodybuilding coach. A million thoughts were running through my mind before I even started training. I was worried about what people would think of me getting involved in bodybuilding because of the negative stereotypes associated with it. But regardless of the concerns, the worries and the pressure, I jumped head first into my new regime. I had 16 weeks to change my body and to showcase my work on stage. I was focused, I was ready and I was determined to take back my life, one training session at a time. Nothing was going to stop me from making this happen, even though I still found myself facing tough obstacles and I still suffered from a crippling lack of self-belief. I had no idea then that one little decision to try something new would change my life. All I wanted at the time was to show myself that I wasn't weak and worthless.

What I discovered as each day passed was that lifting weights was truly empowering. I had never felt so amazing, both inside and out. Every single day, I could see my body changing and it was so exciting. I followed a strict regime, training first thing in the morning, followed by another weight-lifting session later in the evening. My nutrition plan was just as tough, with each meal timed precisely in the day. My entire life revolved around my bodybuilding plan and all I cared about was being successful. Little did I know that I was building myself back up without even realising it.

I was back to waking up early in the morning and I spent all my spare time researching the sport, nutrition and exercise techniques. It wasn't just a case of following the plan set by my trainer.

I wanted to know as much about the process as possible. I wanted to know *why* I was doing certain things – I wanted to know the science and the theory. I have always learned so much better through action rather than just study, so all this new and exciting information was sinking in and it all made so much sense because I was putting it into practice on a daily basis.

But this was still my secret journey and challenge, although I did write about my daily progress and also my new passion for all things fitness on my blog. For the first time I felt like I was totally stripped back, that I was no longer a fraud. Anything I shared was raw and 100% real. I discussed my struggles, my workouts and my food, and the response blew my mind. People were so receptive to my journey and the information I was sharing, especially women. Some of my male audience took a dislike to my new strong, empowered self, but I didn't care. I wasn't trying to look good for some stranger behind a computer. I felt amazing and I no longer strived towards unrealistic body goals or image labels. Also, don't forget that I was just coming out of an abysmal depression, so to be receiving encouraging words from strangers saying that I was inspiring them was really special, so a big thank you if you were one of those people who supported me between January and May 2014 – it meant a lot.

My body was changing significantly each day, and with each day I found myself reclaiming the remnants of my lost self. I even decided to return to study and I took a new business course. Things were starting to come around for me, and fitness was the catalyst. I was back doing things and planning for my future. I had a passion for the world and a renewed sense of self-belief.

Sixteen weeks later, after roughly 784 healthy meals, 150 protein shakes, 224 intense workouts, endless posing sessions and early nights, I found myself a day away from my goal. For weeks, people around me couldn't understand why I would choose to do something so difficult and challenging, with so many sacrifices. But I had fallen in love with testing myself mentally and physically and that rush of exhilaration in knowing few could do it. My confidence was at an all-time high. I even made some new friends along the way. **I had become a stronger woman than I had ever been before.**

I went into my first bodybuilding show with an open mind. I already had a huge sense of achievement even before I stepped on that stage. I wanted to win and I trained every day like I was going to win, but I had no idea that I really would win. I took first place in my category, 2014 Miss Spring Classic over 168cm, and was the proud owner of a giant new trophy. The win was like a fairytale ending, but it was actually just the beginning.

My first bodybuilding show was my turning point back to reality. For anybody who is feeling lost or low, you don't have to take up bodybuilding to find yourself. Just do something new: take up exercise, meet new people, start a blog, sign up for a new course or do charity work. Even if it doesn't work out, it will be the catalyst for change. Drop the excuses and do that thing you have always wanted to do. **Just say yes.** If you want to change, then you have to change something. Think action, not excuses. Think life experiment, not potential failure. Have faith that you will find your way back.

"IF YOU CHANGE THE WAY YOU LOOK AT THINGS, THE THINGS YOU LOOK AT CHANGE."

WHERE I'M AT NOW

It has been two years since I decided to do that first bodybuilding show, and now here I am, writing a book to help other people find out how powerful fitness can be. I've done many more bodybuilding shows in that time. I've even represented Ireland at the IFBB European Championships and I've climbed Machu Picchu for the Irish Cancer Society. My life has not been perfect by any means since then, but sometimes the hardest days are the most significant.

I've discovered that fitness can be a tool for positive change, a healthier mind and yes, a hotter body. It can be a way to vent and shake off some toxic energy and it can even be a future career. It is totally individual and everybody will experience it in a different way. I hope I can inspire you to make it a part of your life, both for health reasons and for the tremendous boost in confidence it will give you.

I've had four serious boyfriends and I learned a lot about myself from each one, but I've also learned that the most important relationship is the one you have with yourself. It's important to take the time to love yourself, to be kind to yourself and to figure out what *you* really want. Surround yourself with people who embrace you for your flaws as well as your positives, but also understand that sometimes things don't work out for a reason. There was obviously a lesson you were meant to learn and it's crucial to identify it, whether big or small. All of these things are a part of your journey to greatness and true self-discovery.

YOUR BODY IMAGE DOES NOT DEFINE YOU

I have learned so much about body image from my days as a lanky dork with a size AAA chest, to my glamour girl days as a model and TV personality criticised daily on social media, and now to my current content self.

The first step towards change is to embrace yourself for who you are today and to stop trying to please other people. You can have the body of your dreams, but you can't look like somebody else. **Strive towards being the best version of *you*.** Invest in yourself and be proud of who you are and what you have to offer. Being yourself is the most unique thing about you, so own it! Be inspired by other women's achievements and actions, but don't try to be them.

> **"HATING YOUR BODY WON'T MAKE YOU SLIM, AND BEING SLIM WON'T MAKE YOU STOP HATING YOUR BODY."**

You need to know that the journey won't be easy. You are going to have bad days and slip-ups; that's called being human. I want you to use your emotions as fuel for the fire, but stop feeling emotional because you aren't perfect. It doesn't matter if you're a size 20 or a size 8, whether you're age 16 or 66, you can always be better. The biggest challenge is to convince yourself of this. I have learned that us women can overcomplicate things, make excuses and sabotage ourselves. Have faith in yourself and stop putting so much pressure on yourself to be perfect, and don't punish yourself for small, insignificant failures.

Your body image does not define who you are as a person. The outside is easy to change; it's your actions that define you and your efforts that people will respect. Life is too short to hate what you have been blessed with, whether you're slim or curvy. Embrace who you are, both inside and out.

I want this book to show you that the tricks to getting fit and healthy are easy – you just have to realise that you can do it. The great thing about fitness is that there is no finish line. There are always ways to improve your diet, change your physique,

get stronger, gain muscle, tone up or become faster. This journey to becoming your new, fit self will be inspiring and enjoyable if you can let go of anxiety and doubt. You can be your own fitspiration if you just try.

I want you to use *BYOB* and fitness to build your confidence and self-worth and hopefully develop a new view on body image. My opinion on body image has totally changed since fitness became my priority. Taking pride in your appearance and having a desire to be better and healthier doesn't make you selfish or self-absorbed. **Focus on health, strength and improvement, and a new body image will follow.**

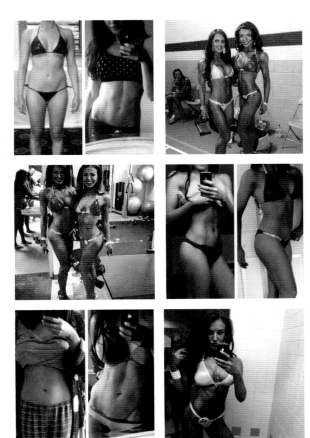

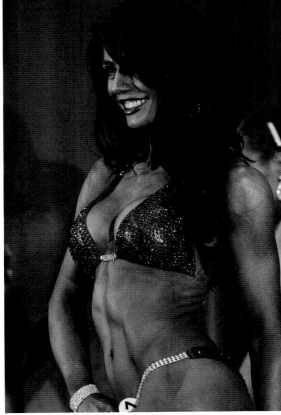

WHAT I'VE LEARNED AND WHAT I HOPE YOU'LL LEARN TOO

- Likes on Facebook and Instagram don't mean success or happiness.

- Taking pride in your appearance, health and body is not shallow.

- Don't compare yourself to other people. Your body and image should be however you want it to be.

- Don't waste your time with toxic situations or people. Nobody has the right to make you feel bad.

- Don't listen to fitness snobs or know-it-alls. There is no one right way to approach fitness. It's a personal thing.

- People will come and go. Learn something from each one and don't forget the people who have helped you along the way.

- It's okay to not be okay. There is a light at the end of the tunnel, I promise.

- Do kind things for other people or do charity work because it's not always about you.

- Be grateful for what you have.

- Be giving, but don't be taken advantage of.

- If you aren't happy with your life, then make a change, even if it's uncomfortable at first.

- If something doesn't work out, it's okay, it wasn't meant to. The hardest situations will make you stronger.

- It's okay to make mistakes.

- Change doesn't mean failure; it's reinvention.

- Set small, realistic short-term goals. Set big challenges and goals for the long term.

- Work hard, be ambitious and dream big.

- Make a bucket list and make it happen. Challenge yourself.

- You are perfect at being you, so be yourself because nobody else can be.

- Never stop pushing for that yes, but also know when to say no.

- Do it with passion or don't bother.

FITNESS AND YOU

Fitness can be so much more than just struggling with your weight. It can be a way to build your strength mentally through physical challenges and it can impact on the rest of your life. I am indebted to fitness for saving me from my darkest and lowest days and for giving me something to have control over when everything else in my life was uncontrollably terrible. Sometimes taking control over your health and nutrition can be the stimulant for taking back control of your life. My journey over the last two years has been filled with many challenges and difficulties, but throwing myself into fitness has basically given me back a purpose. I have learned so much about myself and I've rediscovered a passion for life through getting fit and healthy. I'm not saying things are perfect now. I have my bad days, but I have a new mindset and a new outlet to destress and vent.

"FITNESS IS SO MUCH MORE THAN A WORKOUT."

My main goal now is to inspire you to experience the joy of getting fit. It's a lifestyle that comes with so many rewards. If you use this book as an introduction to the world of fitness, you can see your body change in ways you never imagined possible.

BYOB won't teach you how to become a bikini bodybuilder like me. Instead, it will show you how to take control of your health and nutrition like a bodybuilder does. I

have learned so much from competitive sport, and I want to share some of that same information and those routines with you so that you can get ripped and strong. I don't want you to be a food obsessive or spend your life counting calories. I want you to use the information in this book to have better success with your body goals, because guess what? You can build whatever body you want. If you work hard, train hard and live a healthy life, you will have the body of your dreams.

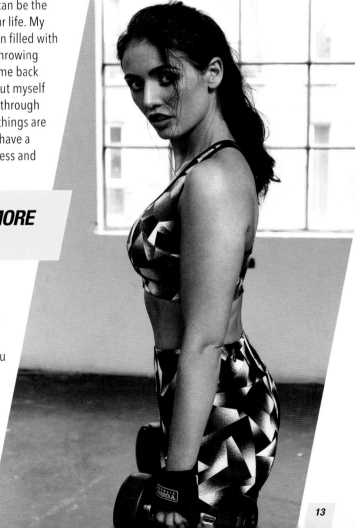

PART 01

THE
BASICS

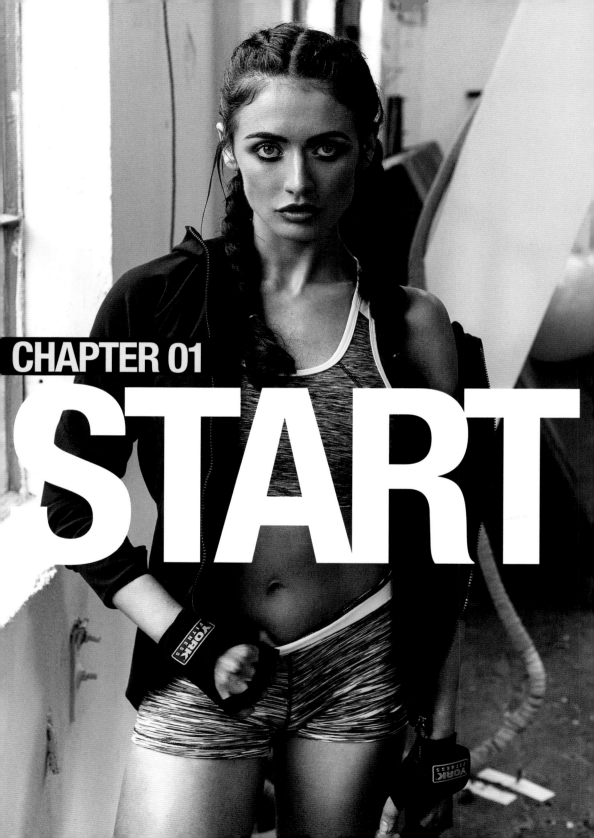

CHAPTER 01
START

In this chapter I will introduce you to the basics. I'll also show you how to analyse your abilities, determine your goals and help you to understand the importance of planning. Are you ready? Let's get started!

THE BASICS

PLAN

If you want to improve your body and your health, you need a plan. Without rules, guidelines and routine, you'll limit your potential success. This doesn't mean you need to plan every second of your day and account for every ounce of oxygen you breathe or every calorie you eat. It means being prepared, having healthy food at your disposal, knowing what your schedule is and locking down when it suits you to work out, making things as convenient for yourself as possible to allow you to get on with your daily life.

Planning means putting your goals on paper and following through with the appropriate action that will help you reach your targets, and Chapter 9 at the end of the book will help you do just that. The other great thing about having a plan is that even if you find yourself struggling or having bad days, you have the information to get back on track without much thought or struggle.

BALANCE

Anybody in the fitness industry will tell you that consistency is one of the most important factors for success, and balance is a key part of consistency. Both are massively important when we talk about making long-term changes to your body. Without balance, you will have a rollercoaster ride with your progress, which is one of the reasons why people give up.

I believe you can have the most success in terms of long-term weight loss and maintaining a healthy body by following the Pareto principle, also known as the 80/20 rule. It's totally pointless to start an extreme fitness plan that you can't maintain in the long term, because all you'll achieve is an unhealthy relationship with your weight and metabolism damage. By living a balanced life, you can enjoy getting fit and losing weight and still allow yourself the things you enjoy, like chocolate or the odd glass of wine. Life is for living and you should be able to enjoy yourself as well as enjoy getting fit and healthy. The main goal with balance is to avoid burning out too soon, overtraining or losing your motivation.

"PUSH YOURSELF, BECAUSE NOBODY ELSE IS GOING TO DO IT FOR YOU."

ACCOUNTABILITY

Just because your mind can pretend you didn't eat that cookie doesn't mean your body can too. **Accountability means taking ownership of your actions.** It's about dropping the excuses, getting out the door and not missing your training sessions. You are 100% in control of your results and your success totally depends on you, so don't cheat yourself and don't lie to yourself. It's okay to slip up, but take ownership of it and be aware of it.

I often hear people say they eat healthy, but they are totally oblivious to all the unnecessary things they put in their mouth throughout the day. I also hear people say they don't have time to train, yet they can find an hour during the day to watch *Keeping Up with the Kardashians*. Sure, there are days when my schedule is totally nuts too, but I make sure I'm up first thing in the morning to get my workout done. Or if I miss that workout, you can be sure that I won't miss it the next day. Be accountable for your actions and be present. No excuses!

NUTRITION

Nutrition is another key to success. **You can't function without food and you certainly can't meet your fitness goals without it.** If you can take control of your daily nutrition and understand it better, you will have much more success with your weight loss and fitness goals.

Food gives us energy. It fuels our minds and our bodies and it's a big part of our daily routine. Food can maximise results, power, endurance and overall health. Eating a nutritious diet can have other benefits too. The World Health Organization and Mental Health Ireland say that it can reduce your risk of disease, improve your skin and hair and promote a balanced mental state.

Your body reacts to the food you put in it, and it will respond positively when looked after with the right nutrition. There's a lot of truth in the saying 'abs are built in the kitchen'. To get a toned, tight stomach, you need to reduce body fat around the midsection, which can be done by manipulating your nutrition plan and by eating a healthy, balanced diet.

Women have always looked at calories as a negative thing, but the truth is that calories are your friend. Calories are just units of energy and your body needs a certain amount each day to

function, let alone if you're looking to get super fit and strong. I'll go into more detail about food in Chapter 4, but for now, suffice it to say that food can be a positive weapon in your weight loss arsenal and that healthy eating doesn't have to be a negative experience.

EXERCISE

Exercise is going to be the outlet for change. It's going to push you and it's going to develop your body and mind. It's going to be the tool that will help you sculpt your body and achieve your goals. You need to start getting excited for workouts and turn it into a fundamental part of your day. Even if you find exercise challenging and difficult, just make it a part of your schedule – eventually it will become second nature and you won't be able to imagine how you lived without it.

> *"GOOD THINGS COME TO THOSE WHO WORK."*

Being fit has immediate benefits. According to the American Heart Association and K.R. Fox, writing in the *Public Health Nutrition* journal, it improves the quality of your sleep, boosts your self-esteem and confidence, helps you be more productive and enhances your mood and mental clarity. Have you ever heard anyone say they regretted doing a workout? No, because usually the hard part is just doing it – once it's done, you feel amazing. Plus by exercising regularly, the Health Service Executive (HSE) says you're maintaining a healthy heart, fighting disease and illness, boosting your immune system, staying slim and keeping fat at bay. Exercise also increases your energy levels and helps to maintain a healthy mental state – **in short, exercise makes you healthy *and* happy**. It's also a great way to be social or get outdoors.

The benefits are just incredible and there are so many of them. It will improve your quality of life overall.

REST AND RECOVERY

It's important to take time out to rest, and by resting I don't mean a night on the tiles. Rest is a vital part of the progress wheel, but a lot of people neglect it. It's one of the most disregarded aspects of improving your body, but I hope that after you've read *BYOB*, you'll start prioritising it. Your body is working overtime from a hectic schedule, stress, anxiety and financial concerns, never mind the added task of getting in shape and maintaining your health. Your body deserves a break!

Making time for rest can actually have huge health benefits, as outlined by the Irish Sports Council, L. Lamberg in *Psychiatric News* and K.D. Tipton and R.R. Wolfe in the *International Journal of Sport Nutrition and Exercise Metabolism*. Not only will it help you maintain a balanced fitness regime and help you avoid overtraining, but it will also help you avoid injury; repair, rebuild and recover muscles; refresh your mind; and replenish your energy levels. The main goal in rest and recovery is to avoid muscle tissue breakdown. **Exercise actually only stimulates your body to change – the real improvements are made during the rest and recovery period.** So to maximise your exercise results, take the time to switch off, eat a healthy and balanced diet to refuel your body and muscles, warm up before a workout, or even try acupuncture, meditation, massage or hydration. It's also important to have a regular sleeping pattern and to get enough sleep every night, which might mean early nights.

REWARD

If you're new to fitness, I want you to start looking at 'bad' food groups in a different way. By utilising reward, you can change your outlook on 'bad' foods and have a more consistent relationship with them and hopefully avoid the dreaded binge eating. I believe it's 100% possible to get shredded and make long-term body changes even with 'bad food' in your diet if you can maintain a balance between good foods and treat foods, differentiate between them and know the right times to eat them.

I know what you're thinking: *This sounds great! I can eat my faves like chocolate, pizza and cake and still get ripped!* Well, no. Unfortunately, it's not that simple. You're going to have to earn your treats through hard work and consistency. You also need to realise that junk food, sugary sweets and processed foods can have a negative impact on your health, but in small doses they can offer some benefits. The definition of a reward is 'a thing given in recognition of service, effort or achievement', so you should acknowledge your efforts and reward yourself accordingly.

> **"REWARD YOUR BODY BY TREATING IT WITH RESPECT AND A HEALTHY LIFESTYLE."**

By using 'cheat meals' in a controlled way, you can maintain your motivation levels and help yourself stay on track with your health and body goals in the long term. I'll talk more about the benefits of rewards in Chapter 8, but for now, just know that you don't have to go cold turkey on chocolate or starve yourself into a bingefest. **Rewarding yourself in a smart way is the answer.**

WHAT I DON'T WANT YOU TO DO	WHAT I DO WANT YOU TO DO
• Criticise yourself too much	• Plan and prepare
• Starve yourself or restrict your diet, or on the flip side, binge eat/drink	• Enjoy getting fit and healthy
• Waste your time and money on fad diets	• Have realistic goals for the short term
• Give up your life, your friends and your hobbies	• Have inspiring goals for the long term
• Think there is a shortcut to success	• Get outdoors – it's free!
• Be tough on yourself when you slip up or worse, quit when it gets tough	• Make better choices
• Say you don't have the time or make other excuses	• Be hardworking and take on challenges
• Be afraid or embarrassed	• Take responsibility for your weight and your health
• Not believe in yourself	• Stop conforming to society's stereotypes
	• Accept that you can't have somebody else's body
	• Love yourself at all stages of the journey
	• Don't accept anything less than amazing
	• Realise that you can have the body of your dreams and that you deserve it

HOW TO GET STARTED

'How do I start?' is always the biggest question and worry for any newbie, but even a pro athlete had to start somewhere. There is no shame in being a beginner. You have every right to be starting a fitness regime and you should be proud of the fact that you are taking proactive steps towards being a better you.

The hardest part is starting and promising yourself that you are going to change. No doubt you've tried some diet in the past that failed miserably or a workout regime that lost its sparkle after a couple of weeks. I can relate, and so can most people. Let go of your past failures and don't carry them into the future. Today is a new day and the beginning of a cycle of success.

As a beginner, I recommend that you start with the basics and don't overcomplicate things. Once you get to grips with the basics and find your rhythm, you can make things a little more challenging. In fitness there are always new ways to push yourself, but for now let's just start, and start slowly.

"SLOW PROGRESS IS BETTER THAN NO PROGRESS."

Of course, it goes without saying that if you are suffering from any serious illness or injury, you should consult your doctor or a health professional before beginning any new workout or diet regime. For now, though, start by making a personal commitment or promise to yourself that you are going to make proactive changes. And not just the typical *Okay, I'll start my diet on Monday*. Start today - start right now! - and get excited about it.

In the beginning, you need to be able to look at yourself and your lifestyle in a constructive and honest way in order to make real change in your life. This involves considering your goals, your capabilities at present, your schedule and also your commitment to planning (Chapter 9 at the end of the book will help you do this). Realistic goals and expectations will help you to have a positive experience. You will always continue to get better and you will always have the option to make things a little bit more challenging - the key is to challenge yourself at your own pace.

DROP YOUR EXCUSES AND LET GO OF THE PAST

Just because previous attempts at getting fit and healthy have failed doesn't mean you're destined to a live a life full of exercise and dieting catastrophes. I'm not saying that your new fit self isn't going to have slip-ups or bad days, because that isn't realistic. What I *am* saying is that you are going to have to work hard and you are going to have to commit to your new lifestyle, but you are going to have a better understanding of what to do when you have bad days and you will pick yourself back up and get back on the fitness wagon. **So say goodbye to your excuses, because that is the only thing holding you back from building the body of your dreams.**

"BE STRONGER THAN YOUR EXCUSES."

WHAT ARE YOUR GOALS?

It's important to know exactly what your goals are so that you can identify what plan and approach you'll need to take. Identifying your goals will give you structure and something to work towards and will also help you monitor your progress. Are you trying to lose body fat, drop a stone, gain muscle, grow a bigger booty, increase speed or simply improve your overall health? Once you've decided what your personal goal is, you'll know which workout plan and diet plan best suit your needs.

"SET GOALS, THEN MAKE THEM HAPPEN."

WHAT ARE YOUR CAPABILITIES?

This is a tough one for anybody to answer, but sometimes it is only in doing so that we can unlock our true capabilities. For example, by signing up to compete in a bodybuilding show, I discovered just how strong and determined I can be, and by climbing Machu Picchu, I discovered how resilient I am. **Each and every one of us is capable of doing amazing things and we all have the potential to be our best.**

"SMALL CHANGES NOW, BIG CHANGES TOMORROW."

Identifying your capabilities will also help you to maintain a consistent fitness regime in the early days of your journey. I want this to be for the long term, and most importantly, I don't want you to quit. Your capabilities right now are significantly different than they will be in a year's time or even in six months' time. Maybe you already exercise quite regularly and have a basic understanding of nutrition, or maybe you're totally new to all this and do no exercise whatsoever. If you're new to fitness, then working out three times a week is a

massive improvement and a realistic beginning to your journey, one that you can maintain until you're ready to further challenge yourself. If you're already a regular fitness bunny, then exercising five to six times a week should be manageable. Have a think about your capabilities, but don't compare your plans and goals to anybody else's.

WHAT ARE YOUR COMMITMENTS AND SCHEDULE LIKE?

If you don't know what your schedule is like, then you can't plan either your nutritional requirements for the day/week or when will be the best times or days for your workouts. For example, if you work 9 to 5, Monday to Friday, then you either need to get your workouts done before or after work or maybe during your lunch break. You need to plan your fitness around your existing commitments. This is about using your time cleverly, being productive and making fitness a part of your life. **Everybody has time to get fit.** There are 168 hours in a week and roughly 56 of those are spent sleeping, so that still leaves 112 hours – use them wisely.

Here are some tips on how to make fitness a part of your life in the long term:

- Take baby steps.

- Make things easy and convenient for yourself.

- Build your knowledge – get curious, ask questions, do research, try a trainer.

- Enjoy eating healthy and exercising.

- Acknowledge your improvements.

- Make long-term goals and plan future fitness challenges.

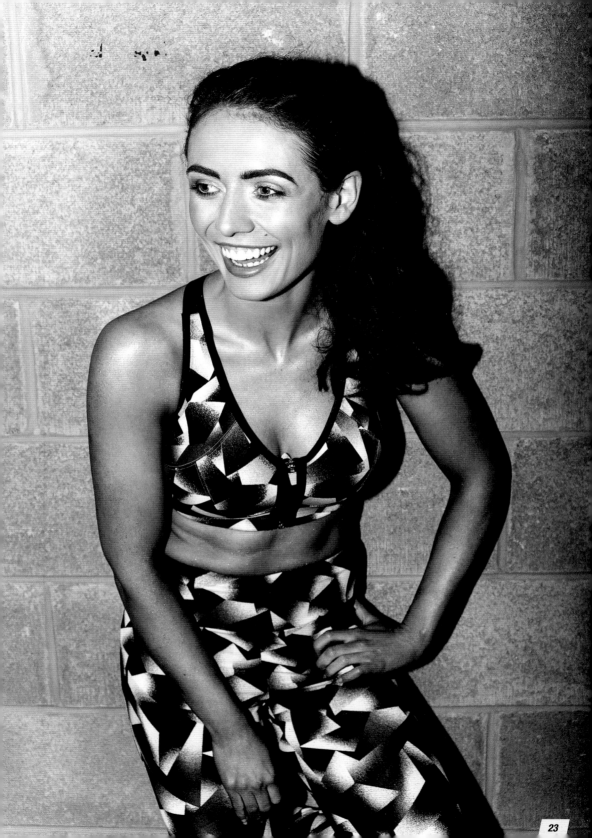

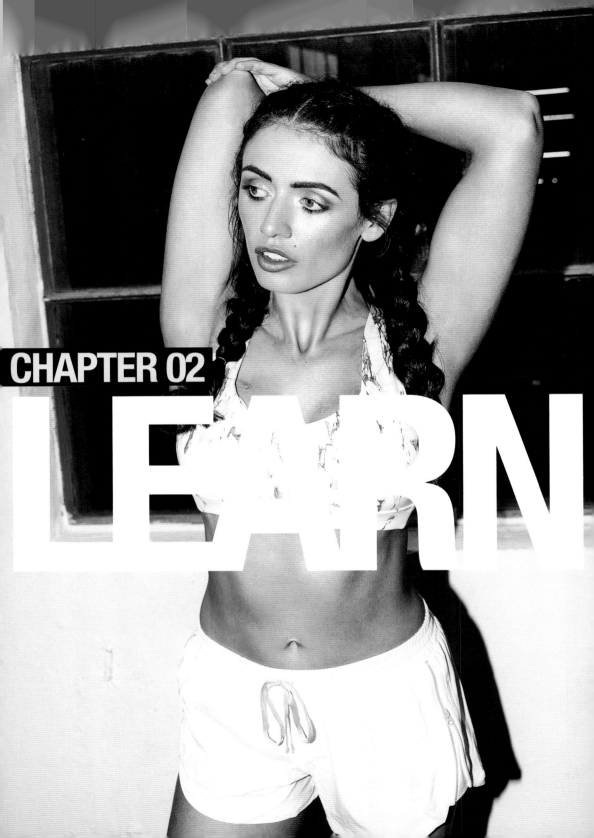

CHAPTER 02
LEARN

Now that you know some of the basics of getting started, let's take things up a notch. In this chapter I'll explain some of the language of fitness, help you to understand how your body works and share some tips for making long-term change. You'll have more success and better progress if you know what things mean and understand how your muscles work.

THE LANGUAGE OF FITNESS

Knowing some of the typical terms used in the world of fitness will help you to be more confident, whether you're hitting the gym or reading an interesting fitness article.

The following lists cover some of the contemporary terms used by fitness heads as well as a tiny snippet of the science and theory behind them. All the information in this chapter is here to help you build your knowledge, which in turn will help you to better understand the workout plans in Chapter 7.

DIET AND NUTRITION

Calorie: A unit of energy.

Calorie deficit: A calorie deficit does not mean eating less. A calorie deficit is created when the amount of food energy (calories) you take in is less than the total calories you use, resulting in weight loss.

Carb cycling: A process where you manipulate the consumption of carbs, rotating between high-carb days to moderate- and then low-carb days. It assists in fat loss and can also be loosely considered as intermittent fasting.

Carbohydrates: Carbohydrates are one of the three nutrients used as energy sources by the body (the others are protein and fat), and carbs are considered to be the most important of the three. Your digestive system turns carbohydrates into glucose (blood sugar) and your body uses this sugar for energy for your cells, tissues and organs.

Cheat meals: The term used to describe a reward meal, which usually consists of food outside of your healthy diet plan. Cheat meals are usually used after a long period in a calorie deficit, normally for fat loss. Using them in a controlled way can help to avoid the negative impact of sustained calorie deficit.

Clean diet/clean eating: A clean diet consist of food like vegetables, fruits, whole gains, lean proteins and healthy fats. A clean diet avoids processed and unhealthy foods.

Diet: The kinds of food a person eats. It can also be a special food plan that a person will follow who wants to lose weight, gain muscle or improve performance.

Diet plan: Guidelines for controlling what you eat.

Essential amino acids: An essential amino acid (or indispensable amino acid) is an amino acid that cannot be synthesised de novo (from scratch) by the organism, but rather must be supplied in its diet. In other words, your body can't make essential amino acids – you have to get them through your diet.

Fasted cardio: Doing exercise/cardio in a fasted state will encourage your body to break down stored fats to fuel your workout. It's a more advanced way to burn fat, but it's not necessary in the beginning phase.

Fat: Fat is a major source of energy in the human diet. Fat has a high caloric content, but a normal intake of fat is essential for your body to function properly. Fat helps your body to absorb certain vitamins, like vitamin A.

Flexible dieting: A process of tracking your macronutrients to achieve a body composition goal.

Fuel: Something that gives nourishment (food).

Glutamine: A hydrophilic amino acid that is a part of most proteins.

Glycogen: A substance deposited in bodily tissues as a store of carbohydrates.

Ketosis: A metabolic process that occurs when the body doesn't have enough glucose for energy. Stored fats are broken down for energy, resulting in a build-up of acids called ketones. A ketogenic diet is also called a low-carb diet.

Macronutrients: Nutrients are needed for growth, metabolism and other bodily functions. There are three major macronutrients: proteins, carbohydrates and fats. *Macro* means 'a large quantity'.

Meal prep: Choosing, measuring and preparing ingredients and food in the hope of achieving maximum results. Food prep/meal prep includes but is not limited to cooking, shopping, budget planning and schedule planning.

Micronutrients: Micronutrients differ from macronutrients in that you need a smaller amount of them. However, they are still essential to maintain overall body health, bone growth and brain function. They are usually referred to as 'vitamins and minerals', which include trace elements like copper, iodine, iron, manganese and selenium and macro-elements like calcium, magnesium and potassium. Micronutrients also include vitamins like A, B complex, C, D, E and K.

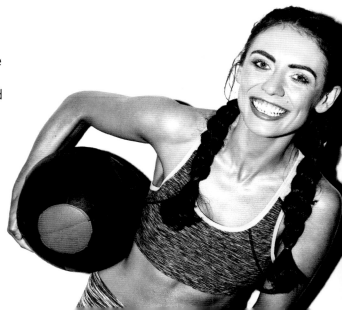

Minerals: Inorganic elements that are essential for the human body to function. They are obtained through food.

Multiminerals: A pill or tablet containing a variety of minerals (dietary supplement).

Multivitamins: A pill or tablet containing a variety of vitamins (dietary supplement).

Nutrition: The process of providing or obtaining the food necessary for health and growth. Also refers to food and nourishment.

Protein: Proteins are one of the three nutrients used as energy sources by the body (the other two are fats and carbohydrates). Proteins are required for the structure, function and regulation of the body's cells, tissues and organs. Meat, dairy, beans and eggs are all good sources of protein.

Refeed: A refeed is different from a cheat meal in that it is usually associated with a less restricted diet plan. The food usually used in a refeed will consist of healthy foods that are already present in the daily food plan. Carb cycling is a clever way to use refeeds to assist in fat loss.

Supplements: A dietary supplement is a product that contains a dietary ingredient intended to add nutritional value to the diet. It can include vitamins, minerals, herbs or botanicals. See Chapter 5 for more information about supplements.

Vitamins: Any group of organic compounds that are essential for normal growth and nutrition. Vitamins are required in small quantities in the diet because they cannot be synthesised by the body.

BODY

Agonist: A muscle whose contraction directly moves a part of the body.

Anabolic: Anabolic is the opposite of catabolic. It refers to the construction phase of metabolism, when body cells synthesise protoplasm for growth and repair.

Antagonist: A muscle that opposes the action of another muscle. For example, the bicep and tricep are antagonistic muscles.

BEE: Basal energy expenditure is the number of calories your body needs to carry out basic body functions like breathing, repair, growing and blood circulation.

BMR: Basal metabolic rate is the number of calories you burn at rest, taking BEE into account.

Body fat: Adipose tissue (body fat) is a normal part of the human body, with a very important function: it stores energy as fat for metabolic demands. Obesity is an excess of body fat, frequently resulting in a significant impairment of health.

Catabolic: Biochemical reactions that break down molecules in metabolism. Molecules may be broken down to gain their energy or to prepare them for disposal from the body. Basically, catabolism is the exclusive provider of energy for the growth and preservation of cells in the body. If you have a high rate of catabolism, your body will break down muscle tissue, which will have a negative effect on the body. You can counteract this process by eating good-quality food, which will assist in muscle growth and avoid muscle loss.

Heart rate: The speed of the heartbeat measured by the number of contractions of the heart per unit of time, typically beats per minute.

Lean: (Of a person) Especially healthy, having no superfluous fat. (Of meat) Containing little fat, non-fatty.

Lean mass: The amount of lean muscle on the body, excluding fat, bones and organs.

Metabolism: Metabolism is a term that is used to describe all chemical reactions involved in maintaining a living state. Metabolism is closely connected to nutrition and the availability of nutrients. Metabolism is broken down into two parts: catabolism and anabolism.

Muscle: A band or bundle of fibrous tissue in a human that has the ability to contract, producing movement in or maintaining the position of parts of the body.

Muscle atrophy: The breakdown of muscle tissue, usually from a lack of physical exercise, though it can also happen due to age and a lack of sleep.

Obesity: A medical condition in which excess body fat has accumulated to the extent that it may have a negative effect on health, leading to reduced life expectancy and/or increased health problems.

Overweight: Weighing more than the normal body weight that is considered healthy for your age or build.

REE: Resting energy expenditure determines the number of calories you burn in a 24-hour period, including activities.

RMR: Resting metabolic rate (similar to BMR) is the number of calories you burn at rest, taking REE into account.

Well-being: The state of being comfortable, healthy or happy.

EXERCISE AND TRAINING

Aerobic: Exercise that improves your body's cardiovascular system, which absorbs and transports oxygen. Cardiovascular exercise like running, jogging and cycling is aerobic exercise.

Anaerobic: Exercise in which oxygen is used up more quickly than the body is able to replenish it inside the working muscle, resulting in muscle fibres sourcing energy from things like stored carbohydrates. Weight training is an example of anaerobic training.

Body weight exercises: Body weight exercises are strength training exercises that don't require free weights or machines. Your own weight provides the resistance for the movement. Sit-ups, pull-ups, push-ups or even TRX (total resistance exercise) are all examples of body weight exercises.

Burn: A gym term to describe the burning sensation you get during intense exercise.

Calisthenics: A form of exercise that consists of gross motor movements, typically without using exercise equipment. This type of body weight training is intended to increase strength, fitness and flexibility.

Cardio: Cardiovascular exercise is any exercise that increases your heart rate.

Circuit training: A form of body conditioning or resistance training using intensity aerobics. An exercise circuit is one completion of all the prescribed exercises in the programme.

Compound exercises: A compound movement or compound exercise requires using more than one muscle.

DOMS: Delayed onset muscle soreness is the pain and stiffness felt in muscles several hours to several days after strenuous exercise.

Drop sets: Drop sets are a weightlifting technique where you perform an exercise and then drop the weight, and continue for more reps until you reach failure. Also called the 'multi-poundage system'.

Exercise: Activity requiring physical effort, carried out to sustain or improve health and fitness.

Flex: A fun word used when showing off or tensing your muscles.

Free weights: A weight such as a barbell or dumbbell that is not attached to another structural device and is raised and lowered using your hands and arms in weightlifting.

Gains: A fitness term used to describe visible progress, including muscle gain and an increase in strength.

Goals: The object of your ambition or effort; an aim or desired result.

High-intensity training (HIT): A form of strength training that focuses on performing repetitions to the point of muscular failure.

High-intensity interval training (HIIT): A training technique where you give 100% effort in quick, intense bursts of exercise, followed by short, sometimes active recovery periods. It's an efficient way to work out and it gets your heart rate up quickly. It can improve your metabolism and athletic capacity and it's also an effective way to burn fat.

High reps: Exercise repetitions over 8 sets. High reps using low weights are a great way to build muscle endurance.

Hypertrophy: Muscle hypertrophy involves an increase in the size of skeletal muscle through a growth in size of its component cells. It's usually as a result of strength or resistance training that stimulates activity in muscle fibres, causing them to grow larger.

Hypertrophy training: A method of strength training intended to induce the fastest muscle growth possible.

Intensity: The amount of physical power that your body uses when performing an activity.

Interval training: Physical training consisting of alternating periods of high- and low-intensity activity.

Isolation exercises: An isolated movement is movement that requires the use of only one muscle at a time. It can also be called concentration exercise.

Leg day: The day of your routine where you train only your legs.

Low-intensity steady state exercise (LISS): A form of exercise, usually cardiovascular, where you maintain a low intensity but keep your effort consistent. By using LISS, your body is encouraged to use fat stores for energy.

Low reps: Exercise repetition under 8 sets. Low reps using high weights are the best option for muscle gain and optimal strength.

Negative (eccentric): The part of an exercise when the weight is lowered.

Negative training: A technique in which you stress the negative phase of an exercise. This style of training is used to condition the body to a new weight.

One rep max: Also called 1RM, in weight training it's the maximum amount of force that can be generated in one maximal contraction.

Plyometrics: Exercises in which muscles exert maximum force in short intervals of time, with the goal of increasing stamina, power, speed or strength. Can also be called plyos or jump training.

Pre-exhaust: As the name implies, you simply pre-exhaust or tire the muscle using an isolated movement before engaging in bigger compound movements, such as donkey kickbacks before deadlifts or squats. Although it's a more advanced technique, it's a great method for muscle activation prior to a workout. I think it's especially useful when training a big muscle group like the glutes.

Progress: Development towards an improved or more advanced condition.

Pumped: A term used to describe the tight, blood-filled feeling in a muscle after it has been intensely trained.

Resistance training: Any exercise that causes the muscles to contract against an external resistance with the expectation of increases in strength, tone, mass and/or endurance.

Rest day: A day spent in rest, especially as an interlude between periods of activity.

Ripped or shredded: Terms used to describe someone with high muscle definition.

Session: The time spent doing physical activity, i.e. a workout session or gym session.

Sets and reps: Sets and reps are the terms used to describe the number of times you perform an exercise. A rep (repetition) is the number of times you perform a specific exercise. A set is the number of cycles of reps that you complete.

For example:

4 sets	10 reps	= 4 x 10
3 sets	15 reps	= 3 x 15
10 sets	10 reps	= 3 x 15

Spot: When a person helps or supports another person with an exercise.

Supersets: An exercise technique where you perform an exercise followed by another exercise with no rest in between. There are two ways to do supersets. One is alternating exercises of the same muscle group, like a bicep dumbbell curl followed by a bicep hammer curl. The other is two exercises for antagonistic (different) muscles, for example chest press followed by lateral pull down for back.

Technique: A way of carrying out a particular task. When talking about fitness, it means the perfect execution of an exercise move.

Train/training: Refers to exercise activity.

Training to failure: In weight training, training to failure is repeating an exercise until you can't continue due to inadequate muscular strength.

Warm up: Prepare for physical exertion by exercising gently beforehand.

Weightlifting: The sport or activity of lifting barbells or other heavy weights.

(Sources: *Cambridge Advanced Dictionary, Encyclopedia Britannica, Encyclopedia of Sports Science, Merriam-Webster Dictionary, Muscle Exercises Encyclopedia, New Encyclopedia of Modern Bodybuilding, Oxford Dictionary of Sports Science and Medicine, Psychology Dictionary* and *Strength Training Anatomy*.)

UNDERSTAND YOUR BODY

Increasing your knowledge is a fundamental part of the proactive *BYOB* process. It will help you break out of your past oblivious exercise cycle, when you may have found yourself doing an exercise move but had no idea why or even what muscle it was working. **If you want to change your body, then you should understand how it works and what it needs.**

This is just a brief and basic introduction. If you want to learn more, check out my suggested list of recommended reading at the end of the book.

The human body: The human body comprises the head, neck, trunk, arms and hands, legs and feet. Every part of the human body is made up of various types of cells, which are the fundamental units of life.

Muscle: A band or bundle of fibrous tissue in the human body that has the ability to contract, thus producing movement in or maintaining the position of parts of the body.

THE HUMAN BODY

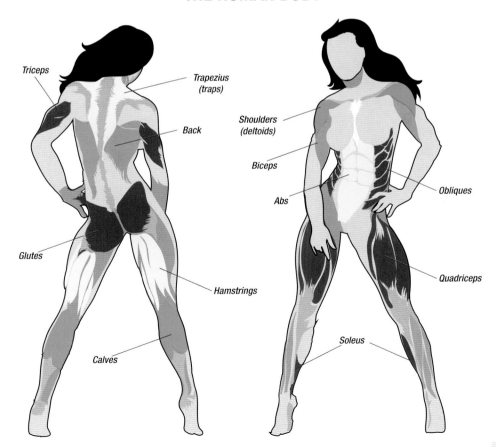

Triceps

Trapezius (traps)

Back

Shoulders (deltoids)

Biceps

Obliques

Abs

Glutes

Hamstrings

Quadriceps

Calves

Soleus

Abs: The rectus abdominis muscle, also known as the abdominals or abs, is a paired muscle running vertically on each side of the anterior wall of the abdomen.

Obliques: The external oblique muscle (of the abdomen) is the largest and the most superficial of the three flat muscles of the lateral anterior abdomen.

Glutes: The gluteal muscles are a group of three muscles that make up the buttocks: the gluteus maximus, gluteus medius and gluteus minimus. The three muscles begin at the ilium and sacrum and are attached to the femur bone.

Calves: The gastrocnemius muscle is located on the back portion of the lower leg. It's one of the two major muscles that make up the calf. It includes the medial and lateral heads.

Soleus: A flat muscle that lies underneath the gastrocnemius. The soleus and the gastrocnemius run the entire length of the lower leg, connecting behind the knee and the heel.

Hamstrings: A hamstring is any of the three tendons contracted by three posterior thigh muscles: biceps femoris, semitendinosus and semimembranosus. The hamstring tendons make up the borders of the space behind the knee. The muscles are involved in knee flexion and hip extension.

Quadriceps (quads): As the name suggests, the quads are a large muscle group that includes the four prevailing muscles on the front of the thigh. It's the great extensor muscle of the knee, forming a large, fleshy mass that covers the front and sides of the femur. The quads are made up of the vastus lateralis, rectus femoris, vastus medialis and vastus intermedius.

Biceps: The bicep is a two-headed muscle that lies on the upper arm between the shoulder and the elbow. Both heads arise on the scapula and join to form a single muscle belly, which is attached to the upper forearm. The biceps are made up of the bicep brachii (short) and bicep branchii (long).

Triceps: The tricep is the large muscle on the back of the upper limb. It is the muscle that is mainly responsible for the extension of the elbow joint (straightening of the arm). The triceps brachii are comprised of the lateral head, long head and medial head.

Pecs: The pectoral muscles (pecs) refer to either of the muscles that connect the front walls of the chest with the bones of the upper arm and shoulder. The pecs include the pectoralis major and pectoralis minor.

Shoulders (deltoids): A thick triangular muscle covering the shoulder joint, used for raising the arm away from the body. There are three parts of the deltoid muscle: the posterior deltoid, medial deltoid and anterior deltoid.

Back: The back is the large posterior area of the human body, rising from the top of the buttocks to the back of the neck and the shoulders.

Trapezius (traps): A pair of large triangular muscles extending over the back of the neck and shoulders and moving the head and shoulder blade, including the rhomboid major/minor, erector spinae, levator scapulae and latissimus dorsi.

(Sources: *Encyclopedia Britannica, Encyclopedia of Sports Medicine and Science, McGraw-Hill Dictionary of Scientific and Technical Terms* and the *Oxford Dictionary*.)

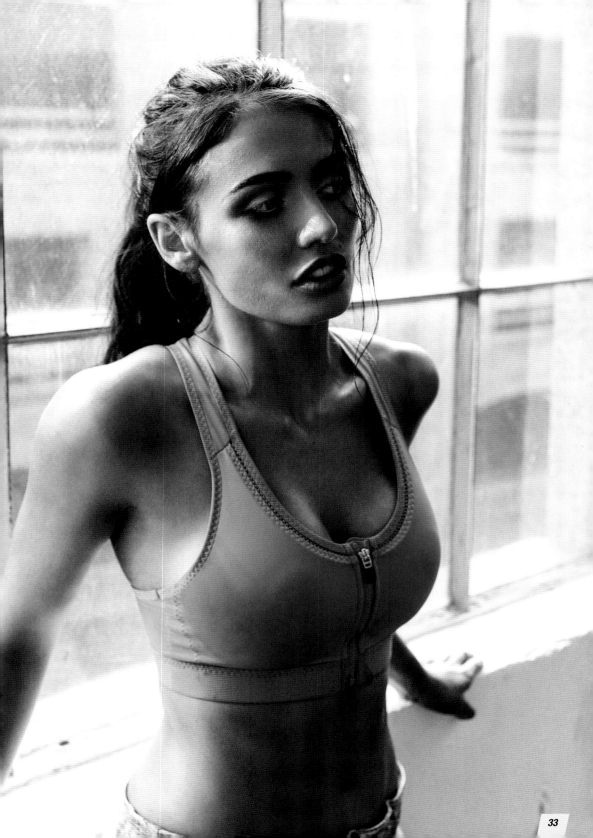

HOW TO MAKE LONG-TERM CHANGE

Have you ever heard the saying that fitness is a lifestyle? Well, if you want to improve your body and maintain your results in the long term, then you will have to adopt this mentality. This is what will stop you from rebounding, yo-yo dieting and losing interest. Everybody wants the six-week body transformation plan to be the turning point of their entire life, and it can be, but only if you have considered what will happen after those six weeks are up. You are changing your life here! **You are about to embark on the journey of becoming strong, fit and powerful.** Restricting yourself and overdoing it in the gym aren't going to help you. Here are some tips for what will.

SET LONG-TERM GOALS

We set goals for other aspects of our life, so why not for our fitness life too? In college we think about our future dream jobs, in relationships we daydream about houses, weddings and children, and when we start a new job we wonder how we can get promoted or get a pay rise. Make fitness a part of your future, just like those other aspects of your life.

This is something I have had great success with, and it's a way for me to stay motivated and excited. Each year I want my goals to become a little bit more challenging, because with each month that passes, my strength and abilities grow, just like yours will.

You probably already know exactly what your short-term goals are. They might include things like weight loss, getting stronger, improving your body overall or increasing your knowledge and understanding of health and fitness. **But have you actively thought about what your long-term goals are?** Are you ready to commit to fitness in the future too?

Here are some ways to plan for your fitness future:

- Book a big holiday.
- Sign up to do a mini marathon, a half marathon or a full marathon.
- Climb a mountain, whether it's Carrauntoohil or base camp on Mount Everest.
- Join a local exercise club, be it cycling, hiking or yoga.
- Sign up for a team sport like rugby, hockey or football.
- Start a fitness blog and share your journey online.
- Take on a physical challenge for charity.
- Go to fitness seminars or talks.
- Commit to maintaining your current results or plan to improve.
- Get your friends and family involved.

The lists in Chapter 9 will also help you to figure out and articulate your goals.

"IF YOU DON'T HAVE A GOAL, THEN WHAT IS THERE TO WORK TOWARDS?"

TAKE BABY STEPS

When it comes to getting fit, there is no secret and no magic pill, just hard work and patience. A slow and steady journey is actually a massive success, and it's a healthy approach to long-term accomplishments and body improvements. You can't become an expert overnight, so just enjoy getting to know your body and making manageable changes each and every day. Taking this approach will stop you from relapsing, binge eating and falling off the bandwagon. **Consistency is king** and it will be the ultimate reason for your long-term success.

BUILD YOUR KNOWLEDGE

Reading this book might be the first step in increasing your knowledge, but it doesn't have to end here. Continue to develop your understanding of how your body works, how food reacts in your body and the latest fitness theories because this will keep you committed and interested. Sports science and theory are fascinating and aren't limited to elites or professionals, so get involved. **There is no limit to the amount you can learn when it comes to nutrition, exercise and health.**

Ask questions, be curious, do some online research, read more books, listen to podcasts and meet up with other like-minded people to talk about your progress and share information with. The list of recommended reading at the end of the book is another good place to start.

ACKNOWLEDGE YOUR IMPROVEMENTS, BIG OR SMALL

You might think that your progress is stagnant and that the changes in your body are insignificant, but the very act of identifying them will encourage you to keep working and pushing forward.

Taking progress photos is a great way to stay motivated and to monitor the changes in your body. These photos can be totally private and for your own assessment. Just take them whenever it suits and compare them every couple of months or even after 12 months. We tend to be our own worst critic, but photos work a treat by providing clear evidence of your progress and success.

And don't neglect your emotional and mental improvements. Do you feel better? Do you have more energy? Are you stronger than you were yesterday or six months ago?

Recognise these improvements and be damn proud of them. Use it is as constant motivation to continue to make even more improvements.

THINK OF FITNESS AS A HOBBY

There is nothing more motivating than committing to a regular hobby. You can't beat the team spirit, competitive feeling and the regular routine it adds to your life. It's also a fun way to commit to a healthy lifestyle for the long term. Bodybuilding is my hobby, but more recently I've taken up hiking. It keeps me on track and has become a normal, everyday part of my life that I love and enjoy.

Find a hobby that you love by trying new things, even if it takes you 10 times to find the one that's perfect for you. You'll have a lot of laughs along the way figuring out what that is, and there is no such thing as a wasted experience.

MAKE THINGS EASY AND CONVENIENT

Let's be real: if something is painful and confusing, then it just won't work. Don't overcomplicate your diet plan or overdo your workout regime. Make sure you maintain a normal social life and still see your family and friends. Schedule in dinner dates, holidays and days off. **The point of fitness is to improve the quality of your life, not to end it.** If you don't strike a balance between everything you love *and* your fitness plans, then you can forget about long-term success.

There are super-simple ways to make this process easy and enjoyable, from having healthy snacks on hand to being prepared and planning in advance.

Here are some tips on how to make health and fitness convenient.

- Take 15 minutes to plan out your week.
- Don't overthink and overcomplicate your plans. Keep it simple and keep it manageable.
- Always be prepared.
- Pick a gym close to your home.
- Train early. We are at our most productive in the morning.
- Always have healthy food in your fridge.
- Chop fruit and veg ahead of time and have them ready to go in the fridge.
- Carry healthy and convenient snacks like nuts, fruit and low-sugar, low-carb protein bars.
- Remember, quality over quantity when it comes to training – 45 to 60 minutes is more than enough time to get your workout done.
- Keep your plans on your smartphone as notes or photographs. It means you have them handy at all times, which makes them easy to follow.
- Pick a motivated gym buddy.
- Make the most of your days off work, which allows for more leeway during your busy week.

ARE YOU READY?

Are you ready to get started? Are you ready to change your lifestyle for the long term, not just for a couple of weeks?

To sum up, you need to:

- Pinpoint what level you're starting at.
- Take into consideration any previous injuries or illnesses that may need professional help before starting.
- Identify what your goals are, both in the short term and long term.
- Plan out your time schedule and when it suits you best to exercise.
- Decide how many times a week you're going to exercise.
- Realise that progress will be slow and steady.
- Have realistic expectations.

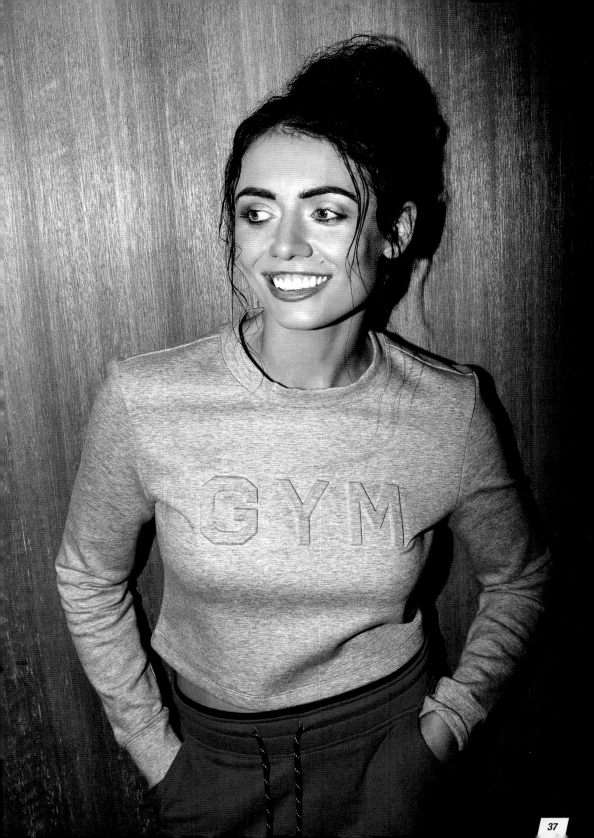

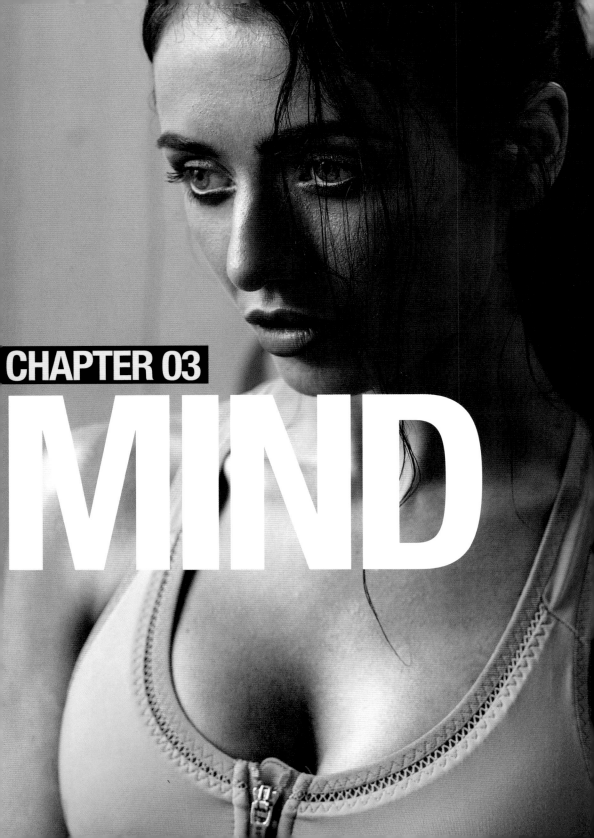

CHAPTER 03
MIND

This book is about positivity and fitness, but this chapter will show you how much of a role your mind plays in your success. Our mind holds so much power over our life and it plays a big part in whether or not we get results. It dictates our mood, it's the reason we stay motivated and it's the source of our success.

The brain isn't a muscle – it's far more intricate in its workings – but **from now on, I want you to start treating your brain like it *is* a muscle**. I want you to train it, and I don't mean by lifting weights with your head! I want you to look after it, I want you to rest it and I want you to get the best results from it. Your mind has massive potential, so why not unlock its strength? Like any other part of your body, the more you challenge it and develop it, the stronger it will get.

THE BENEFITS OF FITNESS FOR MENTAL HEALTH

The Gale Encyclopedia of Neurological Disorders tells us that the brain is the most complex organ in the human body and is made up of more than 100 billion nerves. Its physiological function is to exert centralised control over the other organs of the body. It generates muscle activity and drives the secretion of hormones. Basically the brain controls everything, so it should be your number one priority.

But what is mental health? According to the WHO and the HSE, mental health is defined as a state of well-being. It includes factors like how we view ourselves, how we view the world, how we cope with everyday life and how we feel about others.

Now that you're starting to realise the importance of brain health, you might be wondering how you can improve and strengthen it.

Well, here's the thing: getting fit and healthy actually works in tandem with improving your brain health. It's like a wheel that never stops turning.

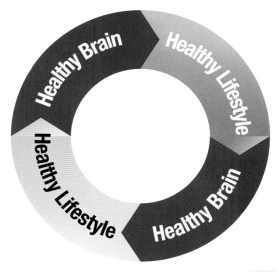

When you exercise, your body releases endorphins, the chemical that is responsible for that happy, exhilarated feeling. It's also responsible for reducing pain. You don't need to start with a lot – according to the Harvard Medical School, exercising three or more times a week is enough to start feeling the mental benefits of exercise and it has been proven to relieve symptoms of mild to moderate depression and unhappiness. It can also help with addiction and improve anxiety. I know it works because it helped me. It allowed me to take control of something when I felt powerless. It gradually relieved my symptoms and gave me back my life.

Investing in the health of your brain is a must, especially if you want to succeed with your long-term body transformation and new healthy lifestyle. By looking after your mind you will be rewarded with a better-functioning body, which in turn will reduce your risk of illness and disease. Plus a healthy mind will improve the quality of your work life, college life, love life, you name it.

We all know what it's like to have our mind run wild with negative thoughts, anxiety and stress. Sometimes life makes it difficult for us to be happy, but then again, sometimes we just make life harder for ourselves. Nobody experiences perfect mental stability every single second of their life. We all have those moments: a job stressing us out, a break-up. I have experienced it too and I can relate, so don't worry if your mind isn't at its best. Even your body image can be a big strain on your brain's health and you can get quite low about it. It can be a vicious cycle, but it's not hopeless. I constantly talk about long-term change, and by investing in your health for the long term, you're also taking care of your brain's health for the long term too. Here are some ways you can improve the health of your brain.

HOW TO HAVE A HEALTHIER BRAIN

EXERCISE

Studies at the Harvard Medical School and the American Psychological Association have proven that **regular exercise does wonders for the brain**, increasing overall function and brainpower. The brain uses the added oxygen in the body as a result of exercise to fix damaged brain cells, increase information processing and memory, and reduce inflammation and insulin resistance. Most importantly, it also improves growth factors within the brain. Aerobic exercise has also been proven to be one of the most effective forms of exercise for the brain, as is exercise that includes additional challenges like co-ordination. A great example of this would be dancing, so why not dance your way to a healthier and stronger brain?

HAVE A HEALTHY DIET

The Royal College of Psychiatrists in the UK states that eating a well-balanced diet consisting of wholesome, nutritious food has been proven to have huge benefits for the brain and emotional stability. Eating a diet that is also rich in omega-3 fatty acids can support better cognitive processes, and research by the UCLA Department of Neurosurgery has shown that by avoiding a diet high in sugar and processed food, you can avoid neurological dysfunction.

According to Mental Health Ireland, the following foods support full brain function and maintain health:

Beef: Normal iron levels in the body are essential for maintaining a healthy brain because iron helps to transport oxygen to the brain, meaning better performance, growth and recovery.

Oats: The main source of fuel for the brain is glucose, which comes from carbohydrates. Oats are a slow-burning carb, which provide brain energy for several hours.

Oily fish: This includes salmon, mackerel and sardines. These healthy fats are super brain food and offer antidepressant and neuroprotective benefits. Bring on the omega-3 amino acids!

Sage: Sage is great for preventing memory loss as a result of acetylcholine breakdown. Why not grow your own sage and cook with it?

Seeds: Both pumpkin and sunflower seeds contain B vitamins and omega fatty acids, which are perfect brain food and will give your brain more energy.

Other great brain foods include eggs, spinach, beans and lentils.

Foods or things to avoid when trying to maintain a healthy mind include:

- Alcohol
- Fried foods
- Highly processed foods
- Refined sugars
- Too much dairy
- Sedentary lifestyle
- Dehydration
- Too much caffeine

BE SOCIAL

A study by O. Ybarra et al. published in the *Personality and Social Psychology Bulletin* in 2008 showed that **being a social butterfly actually increases brain performance and reduces the risk of dementia**. It's time to get involved and get social – your brain will thank you for it. Yes, exercising is a great way to stimulate the mind, but there are many other options too, including reading, meeting up with friends or joining a club.

CHALLENGE IT

If you want a better-functioning brain, then you have to challenge it. The Institute of Public Health in Ireland and the Harvard Medical School suggest that by challenging the brain on a regular basis, you can improve brain function, increase memory and regulate emotions. Things like reading, physical challenges, listening to music, doing puzzles and playing cards are all good examples. But remember, it has to actually be a challenge – if it's easy, then it isn't going to improve anything.

"IF IT DOESN'T CHALLENGE YOU, IT DOESN'T CHANGE YOU."

SLEEP

The Division of Sleep Medicine at Harvard Medical School (yes, there really is such a thing!) has proven that **sleeping over seven hours a night improves brain health – it's not just beauty sleep**! By neglecting your ZZZs you're at risk of a weakened immune system as well as depleted energy levels.

THINK POSITIVE

Thinking positively may sound airy-fairy, but Barbara Fredrickson, a positive psychologist researcher at the University of North Carolina, has shown that it provides long-term health benefits and better brain function. There really is a lot more to positivity than just showcasing an upbeat, enthusiastic attitude. The scientific term for positive thinking is called neuroplasticity, and it basically means that **our thoughts can change the function and the structure of our brain**.

Even if it doesn't come naturally to you, try to look on the bright side because the benefits are there. Having a happy outlook on the world and everyday situations can rewire your brain and arouse positive feelings throughout the body. According to the Harvard Medical School, people who are optimistic also have the added benefit of a longer life span, a reduced risk of depression, anxiety and stress, and they even have stronger immune systems and are less likely to get sick.

GET MOTIVATED!

It's all about that dopamine! You might be asking what the heck is dopamine, or maybe you're already familiar with it because it's linked to things like pleasure and adrenaline. But K.M. Tye et al., writing in *Nature* in 2013, have shown that dopamine is also linked to motivation and that a lack of it can result in mental fatigue and depression.

Dopamine is a neurotransmitter that helps control focus, motivation and productivity. It's made of the amino acid tyrosine, and by getting enough of it in your diet you can increase your dopamine levels naturally and in turn have more drive and motivation.

According to *The Athlete's Guide to Sports Supplements*, foods high in natural tyrosine include:

- Almonds
- Avocados
- Bananas
- Beans
- Chicken
- Fish
- Seeds
- Soybeans
- Turmeric

You can also include it in your supplement stack and try things like:

- Curcumin
- Green tea
- L-tyrosine
- Magnesium

Other ways to increase dopamine include:

- Regular exercise
- Sex
- Sleep
- Sunlight
- Taking on exciting challenges

I'll be honest here – I have bad days and slip-ups, just like everybody else. I'm not some superhuman fitness girl on Instagram you can't relate to. I'm just a normal girl who has found great success with fitness. But I have also been at the starting line, and I still find myself unmotivated every now and then.

People ask me all the time how I stay motivated, and I always say that setting goals and giving myself challenges help me stay consistent. I need both short-term and long-term goals to work towards. I also keep my fitness plan in view on my fridge and on my phone. I use a calendar as a reminder that I'm always one step closer to my goal. I train with friends and I keep junk food out of my kitchen. I also know that nothing happens overnight – having realistic goals is important.

"EVERYONE HAS TO START SOMEWHERE."

That's what works for me, but getting fit is such an individual, personal journey. **There is no one way to approach fitness successfully and there is no wrong way to do it.** But having said that, I find that the best way to stay motivated is to always want to improve and to push yourself. Nobody knows you better than you do, so challenge what you think your limits are. Sometimes staying motivated can be as simple as having a goal, having a plan that will help you meet that goal and then just knuckling down and doing the work. You need to figure out what gets you motivated, and the only way to do that is to try different things.

Here are some useful ways to get motivated, both in the beginning of your journey and for the days when you just need a kick up the butt.

REMEMBER WHY YOU STARTED

Why did you start? Or why do you want to start? Keep that desire to change uppermost in your mind and give it fresh thought any time you feel like you can't do it.

COMMIT TO A FRIEND

There's nothing like a bit of pressure from a close buddy who isn't going to take any of your excuses or nonsense. We can be failures in the privacy and safety of our own heads, but **it's harder to be a failure in front of a friend**. Make a pledge to your besto to exercise together twice a week, or maybe have a weekly check-in to talk about your progress and how you can improve. Support each other and push each other, but don't invite that friend who is a bad influence.

"WHEN TIMES GET TOUGH, REMEMBER WHY YOU STARTED."

MAKE IT PUBLIC

This won't be for everyone, but it's a super way to add a little bit of fire under your feet to continue to progress and follow through with your promises. Share a post on your Facebook, Twitter or Instagram page and tell all your friends and family what your goals are and how you are going to do it. This is a step up from simply getting your best friend involved – this adds a whole other dimension of pressure to succeed. There is a nice element to this one, though, because you'll be surprised by how much your friends on social media will support and encourage you.

SURROUND YOURSELF WITH SUPPORT

Write yourself positive little notes and words of encouragement and keep them in random places like your bedroom, your office or as your screensaver. Surround yourself with like-minded positive, ambitious people who want the same things as you. Seriously, those types of people are contagious and they will help you stay motivated. Follow people online who you think are great, whether it's in the world of sport, fitness or just somebody who shares positive life posts.

DO IT FOR THE HATERS

Use those toxic people in your life – the people who don't believe in you, the negative and pessimistic people – for motivational fuel to succeed. Damn right, girl, prove those people wrong!

GET COMPETITIVE

Nothing beats the rush you get from a competitive spirit, and that exhilaration you get from trying is better than the win itself.

SET A GOAL WITH A TIMEFRAME

Long-term change is a must, but setting goals with a timeline can really give you an extra push. Maybe you know you have a holiday coming up, or maybe you've signed up for a mini marathon. Nothing will keep you more focused or instil a better work ethic than a deadline.

GET DRESSED IN YOUR GYM CLOTHES

Something as simple as putting on your gym clothes will be a positive step towards getting out the front door. Just put them on and see what happens, but you will more than likely end up in the gym. I usually look like a hobbit when I'm training at the gym, but every now and again I'll invest in some stylish gym gear or new trainers. It's a great incentive to get to the gym and give them a whirl. Treat yourself – you deserve it.

AVOID YOUR TRIGGERS

Okay, this is a bit of a cruel one that you're probably going to hate me for, but it's the truth. We all have triggers that can make us horrifically unproductive or lazy. They could be chocolate, friends who love a weekend of binge drinking, your boyfriend, a TV show you're totally addicted to or even social media. Look, I'm not saying you need to ditch your boyfriend or give up chocolate or your Twitter account, but **be aware of the things that distract you and cause you to lose sight of your plan**.

Don't keep junk food lying around your house if you know you go weak at the knees for it. If your friends want to party, do it once a month or once every six weeks, not every weekend. If your boyfriend asks if you want to watch Netflix on the days you train, say no – there's always the weekend. It really is as simple as avoiding the things you think are going to cause a slip-up or that will cause you to make bad choices. They can't tempt you if they're not there.

THE POWER OF WILLPOWER

By now I'm sure you can see how important your mind is in the process of getting fit and that it's going to be one of the keys to your success. **You're going to have to make your brain work just as hard as your body, so it's time to think of your willpower as a muscle too.**

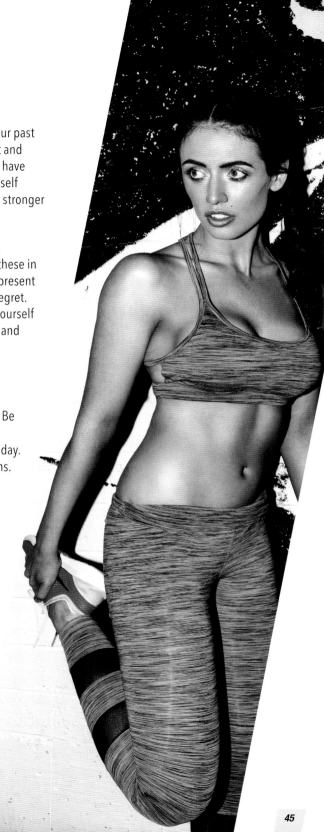

GROW A THICK MIND

A thick mind is kind of like a thick skin. Let your past failures and slip-ups strengthen your present and future decisions. Look at all of the things you have overcome and compare your past self to yourself today. I have no doubt that you have become stronger as a result of hardships.

We all have our own unique life experiences, difficulties and challenges and we all utilise these in different ways to strengthen and mould our present and future selves. Don't live a life based on regret. Come to terms with your past and embrace yourself for who you are today. Love yourself through and through, flaws, quirks, strengths and all.

MIND OVER MATTER

Be present in your life and pull in the reigns. Be mindful and take notice of your energy, your triggers and all the things you do during the day. *You* control your mind and in turn your actions.

CONTROL YOUR EMOTIONS

Easier said than done, I know. Try to manage your stress levels, because high stress almost always translates into mindless, bad choices. Even if you're feeling a little blue, don't give in and let it wreck your plans or goals. Take control of those emotions. Remember, you're in charge.

MAKE SMART CHOICES

Don't be oblivious to your actions. Think about the choices that you have and be clever about them.

Weigh up the pros and cons of every situation and decide if it's the right move or a wrong one. Sure, you could have a takeaway pizza, or you could make your own homemade healthy one. Making small but smart choices like that will help you succeed.

DON'T PROCRASTINATE

Get into a routine. Don't wait until later – get the job done now.

TAKE CONTROL

If you feel like you're going to give in, jump up and make a proactive attempt to take control. Do something else – go for a walk or have a glass of water instead of eating that cookie.

DISCOVER YOUR INNER STRENGTH

I can't really tell you how to unlock your inner strength. The only person who can do that is you. The most important thing is to just do something, but try to go against the grain or overcome that challenge, because **nothing amazing ever happens within the boundaries of your comfort zone**.

I think inner strength means having confidence in yourself, and I don't mean being vain or being the girl who commands the most attention in a room. I mean being confident in yourself and have a sense of self-contentment.

Learn from your past, grow from your mistakes and just love being you. I promise there is strength to be found in that. Surround yourself with people who build you up, who support you and who compliment and acknowledge your achievements. If you waste your time with people who put you

down and make you feel insignificant, how can you ever expect to unlock your true inner strength? Nothing can highlight how far you have come better than the words of somebody else, because sometimes we can't see our own achievements for what they are.

FIND CONFIDENCE THROUGH FITNESS

Fitness is so liberating once you get into it. By starting a new workout plan or taking on a new diet plan, you're already getting out of your own shell and doing something different and positive.

It's hard to feel your best and to be content with what you have because there's always this feeling that we're not quite good enough. The pressure to look perfect, to wear the right clothes, to say the right things, to have flawless make-up or to be toned and tight can be too much sometimes. It's important to take pride in your appearance, but there is nothing quite like that raw, gritty feeling of getting down and dirty in the gym. The sheer freedom of it can be a big boost to your confidence. I know, because it picked me up in my darkest days. If you're feeling down, go work out – it will give you the boost you need.

Lifting some brawn in the gym is utterly empowering and the changes it brings about in your body will build confidence and self-belief. Lifting weights will literally make you stronger, which in turn will make you feel mentally stronger too.

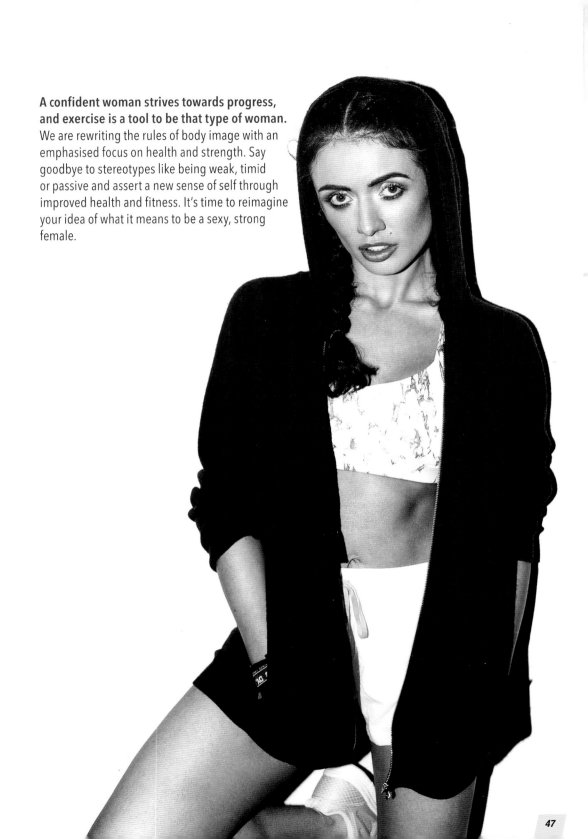

A confident woman strives towards progress, and exercise is a tool to be that type of woman. We are rewriting the rules of body image with an emphasised focus on health and strength. Say goodbye to stereotypes like being weak, timid or passive and assert a new sense of self through improved health and fitness. It's time to reimagine your idea of what it means to be a sexy, strong female.

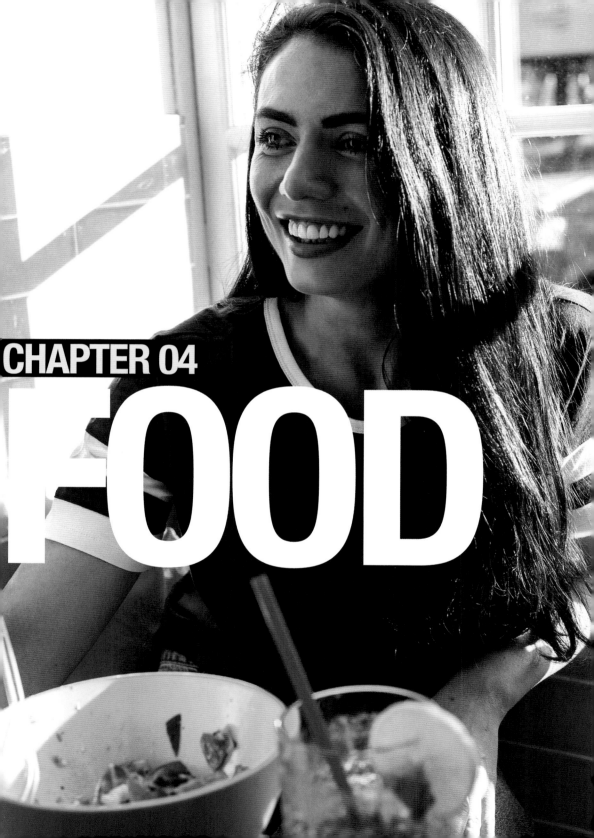

CHAPTER 04

FOOD

I don't want this to be the typical nutrition chapter that just tells you what to eat and what not to eat. In this chapter, I want you to discover *why* you're eating certain foods and what the impact will be on your body. I also want to give you the tools to be confident in your knowledge and to be able to put it into practice.

Before I got into fitness, I thought eating healthy meant eating toast and a bowl of cereal in the morning, having three meals a day and not eating after 6pm. If I wanted to lose weight I restricted myself as much as possible because I thought starving myself was the way to do it. Not surprisingly, that plan only ever lasted a few hours and typically ended with me raiding the entire contents of my kitchen. But now I understand why I could never improve or succeed – I didn't have the right information. **Information is king, and it's up to you to get yourself informed.** Visit a dietician or nutritionist, jump online, download the latest app or read a magazine to get information on good food, examples of diet plans and nutritional value calculators. There's no excuse to be uninformed.

We eat food every single day of our lives, so in theory we should all be pros at it. The reality, though, is that most people only have an obscure understanding of how to have a healthy, balanced diet as well as how to eat for your goals. Not everybody wants the same thing, so nutritional plans are not one style fits all. I know from experience that certain foods don't agree with me and I simply don't want to eat some foods – I don't care if mushrooms are healthy, I just don't like them!

Now don't go using my hatred of mushrooms as an excuse to say 'I don't like healthy food, so I'm not going to eat it'. I mean, who doesn't want to eat Nutella all day? But you have to suck it up and embrace healthy food.

YOU ARE NOT FAT – YOU HAVE FAT

So let's talk woman to woman here about food. If we're honest, most of us have a pretty bleak past relationship with food that would make our love lives look simply rosy. Trust me when I say that I understand and I have been there. I well remember the dark days of demolishing an entire tub of Ben and Jerry's without my stomach even registering the food as being eaten. To this day I will confess that I'm no stranger to the odd bingefest or bad day, even sometimes an entire bad weekend, because guess what? I'm human and it happens. The difference, though, is that now I'm aware of what I'm doing. I know I'm splurging. I'm mindful and conscious of it rather than just shovelling food into my mouth willy nilly. I have also stopped beating myself up after a bad day. If I gain a bit of weight, who cares? It's just body fat and I know I have the tools and information to lose it again.

I read a fantastic fitness quote about two years ago. I thought it was brilliant and decided to share it, and to date it's still my most popular blog post:

YOU ARE NOT FAT. YOU HAVE FAT. YOU ALSO HAVE FINGERNAILS BUT YOU ARE NOT FINGERNAILS.

It's really powerful and it perfectly explains exactly what I'm trying to say. Body fat is something that you can gain or lose. It doesn't have any power, it doesn't symbolise your soul and it doesn't define you as a person. The same goes for somebody who may be insecure as a result of being naturally very slim. Neither of these issues should cause sadness, anxiety or frustration, because the good news is that you can do something about it. **I have learned that working towards the body of your dreams isn't about being perfect, it's about trying.** It's about consistency, heart, taking responsibility and dropping the excuses.

"YOU HAVE TO EARN A GOOD BODY."

EAT REAL FOOD

When thinking about what foods you should be eating, the most important thing to remember is to **eat** *real* **food**. And when I say real food, I don't mean food that is labelled *natural* or *low fat*. I mean genuinely real food: food that comes from the ground or from a tree. Real food usually doesn't come in a microwavable package or jar, and it definitely isn't highly processed or loaded with sugar and chemicals. Real food is 100% natural – not because the package says it's natural, but because it still has it original integrity and nutrients.

People are always looking for secret foods and fads to help them lose weight and get fitter, but if you eat real food, you genuinely can't go wrong. It's

about eating the foods we are designed to eat and simplifying things that we insist on complicating. The WHO, the Nutrition and Health Foundation of Ireland and the Irish Nutrition and Dietetic Institute all tell us that by eating a diet consisting of lean meats, fresh vegetables and healthy carbohydrates, you will improve your physique, lose fat, gain lean muscle, improve your health and increase your energy levels. This is the most important aspect of your fitness plan and your body will see the biggest changes from it.

FOOD IS FUEL

Healthy eating isn't just about a six-week plan to lose as much weight as possible. It's about embracing and enjoying healthy food every single day for the long haul. By building your understanding, you can also use food as a tool to help you reach your body goals and fitness ambitions. **Start thinking of food as fuel and thinking of calories as your friend, not your enemy.** Food should be enjoyed, but you need to realise the difference between food that is going to help you function and look better and food that will only do the opposite.

In *BYOB*, treat food is called a treat for a reason – you should only reward yourself with it every now and again. I'm not saying you need to stop enjoying your favourites, but it's time to let go of the emotional connection you might have with some foods and take control over your eating habits. Enjoy healthy food and eat it regularly, then have a well-deserved and hard-earned treat once in a while.

And speaking of eating regularly, that's really important too. The Medical Research Council and Dr Sandra Drummond from Queen Margaret University College in Edinburgh recommend that we eat four to six small meals a day instead of the typical three. In addition, the *American Journal of Clinical Nutrition* and the National Institutes of Health say that eating little and often throughout the day has many benefits. It stabilises blood sugar levels over the day, meaning you will be less likely to make bad food choices, and it will keep your cravings at bay. This approach lowers insulin resistance too. Your body will respond positively to the routine, so get into the habit of eating moderate portions and more often.

When it comes to food, the biggest pitfalls are usually being lazy, unprepared or unimaginative. A lack of knowledge can also really hold you back. It's crazy how little most people know despite how much information is at our fingertips. But the truth is actually quite simple: **when it comes to diet, there are no shortcuts, just real food and realistic diet plans that work with your life**. You can make delicious, healthy food that tastes amazing, you can make healthy versions of your favourite naughty treats and you can even use treat food to help you lose body fat.

In this section of *BYOB* I'm going to give you a crash course in nutrition. You are going to eat like an athlete, be prepared like a champ, be informed like an expert and look like a goddess. It's time to use your new knowledge to help you get the body of your dreams.

FOOD IS YOUR FRIEND

Food is not the enemy. Sometimes I think it's our own minds that are the enemy. Who controls a car? You do. Who controls what you wear? You do. So who controls what you eat? You do. What you eat or how much you eat doesn't define you as a person. It won't make any difference to the contribution you make to the world and it won't stop you from doing amazing things. **It's just food. It isn't out to get you or ruin your life.**

In fact, food is your friend. Food is the reason you're able to grow curvy muscles. It's the reason you have energy. It's the reason you don't get sick and it's the reason you're able to live your life to the fullest. And the more good food you eat, the better you will look and the better results you will get from your workouts. Then, when you get that well-deserved bar of chocolate or double-decker burger, you'll really appreciate it. That's why it's called a reward. The only enemy you need to banish is the person inside of you who is holding you back.

WHAT ARE THE BENEFITS OF A GOOD DIET?

Food is the source of energy for your body that allows it to function, recover and grow. Food supplies your body with the vital nutrients that you need to survive, but the benefits of a good diet go far beyond that.

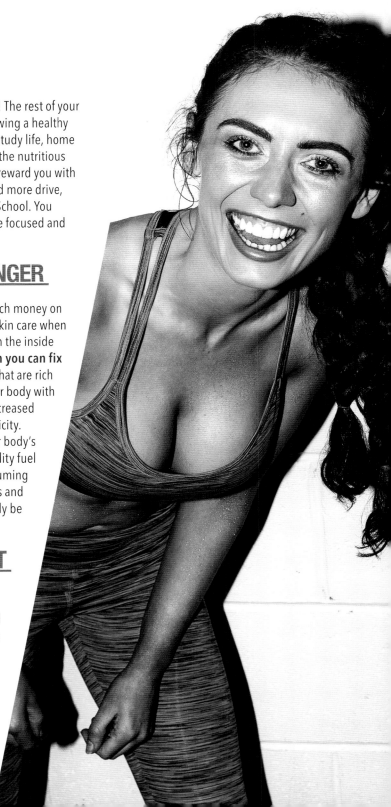

YOU'LL KICK ASS

And not just in the world of fitness! The rest of your life will improve as a result of following a healthy and balanced diet: your work life, study life, home life, the works. Your body will love the nutritious food you offer it and in return will reward you with bags more energy, better focus and more drive, according to the Harvard Medical School. You will even find yourself feeling more focused and organised.

YOU'LL LOOK YOUNGER

It's crazy that women spend so much money on make-up, beauty treatments and skin care when they don't invest in their body from the inside out. **Why hide the problem when you can fix it?** By consuming delicious foods that are rich in nutrients, you are providing your body with internal anti-ageing properties, increased immunity and improved skin elasticity. Did you know that your skin is your body's largest organ? It needs a lot of quality fuel to function at its best, but by consuming lots of different nutrients, minerals and antioxidants, your skin will naturally be glowing and fresh.

YOU'LL GET TO EAT MORE

The good news is that healthy food choices tend to have fewer calories than junk food, which means you can eat more of it – and who doesn't love to eat? Plus the more healthy food you eat, the more you *want* to eat it. I've noticed that the more healthy food I eat, the better I look.

That being said, I always stay within the guidelines of my body requirements, even if I'm not counting every last calorie. It's much harder to overeat on a healthy diet than on a diet full of junk food.

The bad news, though, is that you can still gain weight even if you eat a very healthy diet, so you do still have to watch it. **There is one law when it comes to weight gain: if you eat more calories than you burn, you will put on weight.** For example, if your body maintenance level is 2,000 calories a day but you consume 2,500 calories, even if it's healthy food, then your body will store it as fat because it has no other use for it.

YOU'LL GET TO SAY SO LONG TO CRAVINGS

We all get them, and when they hit, they hit us hard. Dr Bernard Jenson and nutritionist Shona Wilkinson have outlined that cravings happen when your body is lacking in nutrients. For example, if you find yourself craving chocolate, you could be lacking in magnesium, while a longing for fatty foods could mean a lack of calcium. But you can counteract the urge to binge by consuming the right foods. And as an added bonus, after a while, you'll notice that your desire to indulge in sugary, heavy foods will have disappeared.

Here are some things to look out for to help you avoid giving in to cravings.

Have you eaten enough during the day? Maybe you missed out on meals or skipped breakfast.

Eating healthy food regularly throughout the day will help you avoid unwanted cravings.

Do you have a lot going on? If your stress levels are high or you're feeling extra emotional, it can cause cortisol levels to spike and in turn your body will seek rewards. Put down that tub of ice cream and get outdoors, do some exercise and take proactive steps against emotional eating.

If you genuinely can't get chocolate out of your head, at least make a better choice by having dark chocolate. Dark chocolate has fewer carbs, half the sugar and a range of nutritional benefits over its milk counterpart. For example, a study on cocoa and cardiovascular health published in the *Circulation* journal in 2009 says that dark chocolate supports blood vessels, meaning better blood flow, and reduces blood pressure – in small doses, of course! Or if you really want a burger, make a healthier homemade one. By making better food choices, you can save yourself so many extra unwanted calories. You'll also curb the craving and keep yourself on track with your diet plan.

YOU'LL BANISH THE BLOAT

Bloating isn't a result of the amount of food you eat, but rather the *type* of food you eat. Certain foods will cause your stomach difficulty and in turn you'll find it hard to digest them, and boom, bloated belly. Clean eating gives your tummy a break. But if you are suffering from bloating or water retention, the US's National Institutes of Health suggest you give these tips a try.

Increase your potassium: Potassium helps to balance and circulate fluid around the body.

Drink plenty of water: Drinking plenty of water throughout the day will help flush your body of toxins and improve constipation.

Drink herbal teas: Many herbal teas have natural diuretic and anti-bloating properties. Try peppermint tea, green tea, nettle tea and dandelion tea.

Avoid overeating: Try to eat until you feel satisfied rather than to capacity. Your body will tell you exactly the point at which a meal is enough. Don't eat food just because it's on the plate.

Eat asparagus: Asparagus is a natural diuretic and can help relieve water retention. It's also one of the most nutritious foods and is full of antioxidants.

Eat more fibre: Fibre is an undervalued but essential component of the healthy food wheel. Fibre helps your body remove waste and unneeded nutrients. Taking roughly 20 grams of fibre every day can improve your colon health and therefore aid in better digestion.

YOUR CLOTHES WILL LOOK BETTER

Maybe it's just me, but there is nothing worse than when your jeans hug your ovaries with a near-death grip, or as my sister says, stuffed sausages. Clean eating will help you fight the bulge and make your clothes look like they are brand spanking new.

YOU'LL SLEEP BETTER

Is there anything more annoying than getting into bed and not being able to sleep? Or even worse, a broken night's sleep, when you find yourself waking up at the sound of a water drop? The Academy of Nutrition and Dietetics has shown that a lack of minerals has been associated with insomnia and bad sleeping patterns. By eating a diet rich in minerals, you'll be tucking in for a better night's sleep, and a girl needs her beauty sleep.

YOU'LL LOSE WEIGHT

It's true that you can shed a lot of excess body fat by following a good nutritional plan, even without doing much exercise or activity. But it's also true that **you can't out-train a bad diet**.

YOU'LL SEE THE RESULTS

So to sum up, by eating healthy, nutritious foods, you can expect to see an instant increase in energy, better digestion and reduced bloating. In the following weeks you should also see further reduced water retention and bloating and you should have lost a noticeable amount of body fat at a steady, consistent rate. Your cravings will have stabilised and even your skin will be looking fresher. In the long term, you can expect to hit your body goals and to be in a position to maintain them and think about future goals.

HOW TO BREAK THE BINGE–PURGE CYCLE

Listen up, ladies, it's time to break that vicious and mentally draining cycle of diet and fail, diet and fail. The binge–purge cycle is the act of repeatedly losing then gaining weight. It's also called yo-yo dieting.

This isn't just a case of falling off the bandwagon or a *so what* mentality. Analytical Research Labs in the US says that it actually has serious long-term health effects that will make you gain more weight in the end. We have already talked about the importance of planning and being aware of calorie intake, but to break the yo-yo cycle you have to think in a realistic and balanced way. **It's not**

about restricting yourself. It's about eating the amount of food that your body needs, allowing yourself a few guilt-free rewards and not eliminating any major food groups. It's about consistently giving your body and mind what they need. The main goal is to avoid undereating as well as overeating.

One of the worst aspects of the binge–purge cycle is the mental punishment you experience during the restriction phase and then again in the binge phase. It's a toxic mental cycle, but you can break

maintaining a life full of rewards, or a short-term fix that requires you to restrict your diet, feel hungry and fight cravings while only delivering temporary results that quickly disappear, and what's more, leave you larger than when you started. Which one sounds better? It's plain to see that a long-term lifestyle approach offers maximum results.

So how can you avoid getting stuck in the binge–purge cycle? Read on to find out.

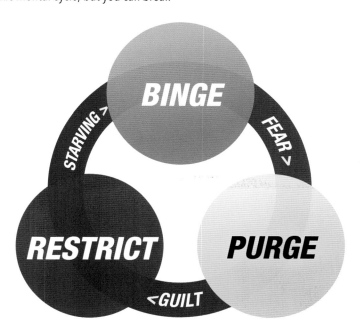

out of it with a new mentality towards getting in shape. By approaching fitness on a long-term basis, you will slowly and steadily work your way towards your goals and avoid the quick-fix solution, which simply doesn't work.

Let's weigh up the options: a consistent, well-maintained body that looks great all year round as you make constant progress while still

YOUR DIET SHOULD SUIT YOUR LIFESTYLE

If your exercise and diet plan are completely at odds with your daily tasks, be it work, college or motherhood, then you are destined to fail. Your plan should work around your life and slot in harmoniously with it. Getting fit should be a positive experience, not a painful one.

GIVE YOURSELF GUILT-FREE TREATS AND A SOCIAL LIFE

What's the point of having a super body if you never get the chance to have fun and show off your results? Use the reward system to give yourself a well-deserved treat and a mental break. Yes, junk food is bad for you, but every now and again everybody deserves a treat without beating yourself up about it. Sometimes you slip up as well, and that's okay too. One little slip-up doesn't have to result in a week of binge eating and mental torture. By allowing yourself regular treats and fun, you will be able to make this a much more long-term change and avoid yo-yo dieting.

SET REALISTIC GOALS

Everybody wants that quick fix, but it doesn't exist. Being patient and having a realistic goal like losing one pound a week is a great way to ensure long-term success.

"STRIVE FOR PROGRESS, NOT PERFECTION."

NEVER RESTRICT YOURSELF

Today's fit woman knows that a starvation diet is a fool's game that doesn't reflect the image that a true health advocate will project. A strong, healthy woman eats often, has control over her eating habits and knows that a restricted diet will hold her back from her fitness and body goals. Respect your body and invest in it, not neglect or punish it.

So what happens when you starve yourself and restrict your diet? Firstly, it's inevitable that it will be followed by a junk food binge, which completely defeats the purpose. The second major problem is that it totally messes up your metabolism and hormone levels as well as your insulin and glucose resistance, which has been shown in studies by L.A. Jason et al. (2003), R.M. Anson et al. (2003), E.C. Westman et al. (2007) and M. Rosenbaum et al. (2008). You will also find yourself becoming more sensitive to food, meaning quicker weight gain, and you will develop potent bad breath. You're reading this book so you're obviously interested in getting more toned, gaining muscle or getting stronger, but restricting yourself on a starvation diet is a guaranteed way *not* to make these goals a reality.

Starvation and restriction are catabolic, which means it's an activity that doesn't support muscle and strength growth. So if you're looking for a toned, tight tummy and a big, voluminous bum, starvation is the wrong way to go about it. You need to look after your muscles with consistent and constant fuel through food to give you the energy to perform well in the gym. By reducing your calories significantly you may lose body fat in the short term, but you're also guaranteed to lose lean muscle mass.

Think about it: ruined metabolism, hormone imbalance, food sensitivity and reduction in lean muscle – everything a fit girl hopes to avoid. You need to eat enough calories with all the right nutrients to support body improvement.

I'VE HAD A BINGE MEAL OR BINGEFEST, HELP!

Step away from the binge and get into a new way of thinking. Everybody slips up. It happens and it isn't the end of the world. It isn't going to totally ruin your improvements, because remember, this is a slow and steady process that will take time and patience. Expect that slip-ups are bound to happen and stop beating yourself up about them. Now that you know the damage binge eating causes from weight gain, messed up hormones and reduced metabolism, hopefully you'll be less likely to binge anyway.

But mistakes do happen and knowing how to deal with them is important too:

- Remember that you're allowed rewards and cheat meals, so appreciate them and make the most of them.

- By following the guidelines and by eating enough calories, you should avoid the desire to binge. Never restrict your diet because it could result in a bingefest.

- Don't beat yourself up about it. Mental torture won't make the situation any better. In fact, it will just cause you further distress, which may encourage you to keep binge eating. Forget about it and move on.

- Use exercise to combat the high level of calories and reduce the damage. Just get up and go.

FOOD INTOLERANCES

Being body conscious means eating consciously, like not eating when you're full or waiting until you are genuinely hungry to eat, which is your body telling you it's time to fuel up. Listen to your body, because it will tell you exactly what you need.

It's important to be body conscious and to eat intuitively, but you also need to know that **there is a difference between having a food allergy and a food intolerance**. Safe Food Ireland and Allergy UK say that a food allergy is more of a reaction that is caused by the immune system, which also results in severe symptoms. A food intolerance isn't as simple to identify. A food intolerance isn't life threatening but can cause serious discomfort and pain. Symptoms can include bloating, constipation, diarrhoea or even skin problems and breakouts.

For example, I now know that some cruciferous vegetables like broccoli and Brussels sprouts (which are my favourites) can cause me to bloat. I by no means have an intolerance to them and I still eat them regularly, but when I'm being very strict with my diet, I will switch them up and eat more spinach and asparagus instead.

If you find that certain foods give you severe constipation or even breathing problems, you may have a food intolerance, which is worth seeking professional help for. If you think you have an issue with a certain food or maybe you just want to find out what works best for you, keep a food diary and write down what food you eat and how it made you feel, especially one hour after you ate it – look out for bloating and gas in particular. This is a great way to pinpoint any issues.

FOOD MYTHS

Despite having more information available to us than ever before, there are still so many misconceptions about food. Here are a few of the ones that are still stubbornly sticking around.

MYTH: FAT IS BAD

Poor fats, they have got a bad rap. Healthy fats like olive oil, avocados, eggs and even salmon are a super – and necessary – part of our diet. The new consensus is that the real enemies are saturated fats, refined sugars, fructose and processed meats, which all cause visceral fat and other health issues. Healthy fats, however, are an important part of our diet. According to the Mayo Clinic, they should make up 20% to 35% of your daily intake.

MYTH: TOO MANY EGGS ARE BAD FOR YOU

Yes, it's true that egg yolks are high in fat, but remember, at least 20% of your daily diet should be made up of healthy fats. It boggles my mind that people who eat a diet full of sugar and highly processed junk worry about eating too many eggs in a week. You are in more danger of heart disease and high cholesterol from eating cupcakes and takeaways. I say bring on the eggs!

MYTH: CARBS MAKE YOU FAT

Carbs are not the enemy and they are not the sole reason for fat gain. **Overeating *any* food group will pile on the pounds, no matter what food group it is**. Carbohydrates are an essential part of your diet and you should think of them as a positive. And don't confuse carbs with junk food. It's true that highly processed junk food is high in carbohydrates, but it's also high in sugar, which offers no nutritional value or positives. Good carbohydrates like sweet potatoes, white potatoes, rice, couscous, beans or quinoa are packed full of benefits that can help you look and feel better. Junk food does the opposite.

MYTH: EATING AFTER 6PM MAKES YOU FAT

This is another myth. **Calories have the same value throughout the day and never change.** I sometimes eat as late as 10pm while still being the proud owner of a six pack. The key is to eat light meals late in the evening that won't hinder your sleep, and it goes without saying that you should avoid sweets and junk food late at night too. Ideally you should eat every two to six hours; after six hours without food, your body goes into starvation mode. Again, the only way to gain body fat is by overeating and underexercising. The time at which you eat your meals is irrelevant.

MYTH: YOU CAN UNDO A BAD DIET WITH EXERCISE

Some people like to think they can eat whatever they like and that exercise will balance out the damage. This simply isn't true. **If you have an unhealthy diet, all the exercise in the world won't cancel it out.**

Think about it this way: it will take you roughly 50 minutes of exercise to shift a single Mars Bar. That's an entire workout to compensate for one small treat. Instead, why not eat nutritious food and lots of it – good food that your body will use as energy – instead of constantly trying to cancel out the bad food? You will make your life easier and you'll get the best results from your workout if you eat less junk.

MYTH: FAD DIETS WILL GIVE YOU RESULTS

Fad diets are everywhere and they are so annoying, whether they promise you'll have a sculpted six pack in a month or you'll lose a stone in six weeks. We've had the Atkins diet, the baby food diet, juicing diets, detox diets and high-fat diets, not to mention all the products that promise to be the miracle cure you've been searching for.

Some of these approaches will deliver on their promise, but the big issue is the timescale. They usually operate within a short-term turnaround at the cost of a low-calorie diet or by neglecting a major food group, like carbs. Would you be so enthusiastic if you were told you'll lose a stone in six weeks, but you'll gain an additional half a stone on top of that six to eight weeks after you quit the diet, meaning that in the long run you'll actually end up bigger than you were when you started? Doesn't sound so appealing now, does it?

Restricting your diet is a no-no, plain and simple. The National Health Service in the UK says that it will only lead to long-term weight gain and health risks like anaemia, tiredness, muscle loss, gallstones, metabolism damage and heart problems. Be smarter than those stupid adverts and realise that a balanced diet that includes *all* parts of the food wheel are necessary for your body to function. Forget the meal replacement shakes and waist trainers and start eating real food that comes from the ground, grows on trees and isn't made in a laboratory test tube.

MYTH: USING A MICROWAVE REMOVES NUTRITION FROM FOOD

This is an interesting one because a lot of people are anti-microwaves, and I believed this too for a long time. But the truth is that **overcooking food, no matter what medium you use to cook it, results in a loss of nutrients**. Overcooking using the oven or grill has the exact same results as overcooking using a microwave. Cook your food with care and don't zap away all of the goodness.

MYTH: GLUTEN-FREE FOOD IS BETTER FOR YOU

Gluten is a naturally occurring protein in wheat, barley, rye and other grains, and unless you are intolerant to it, are a coeliac or suffer from non-coeliac gluten sensitivity (NCGS), you can include it in your diet and still get in great shape.

Gluten-free food has become very topical and trendy of late, but it's often just another advertising attempt to convince people they are eating healthier. The irishhealth.com website says that roughly 1% of the population suffers from coeliac disease, which translates into seven in 1,000 people. If you're not in this group, then don't waste your time worrying about gluten-free food. If you think you have any issues with gluten, you should of course talk to your GP about it.

MYTH: MILK IS THE BEST FORM OF CALCIUM FOR YOUR BONES

This can be quite controversial, since dairy is such a large part of everybody's diet, but my personal opinion is that we should only consume a small amount of dairy every day. Milk is a fattening agent for infants, and animals will stop drinking milk at any stage up to one year. So why do we drink milk as adults, never mind from another species? Personally, I have seen a lot of benefits from reducing my dairy consumption.

MYTH: ALL SMOOTHIES AND FRUIT JUICES ARE GOOD FOR YOU

It's tempting to buy a premade juice or smoothie in the hopes that it's healthy, but unfortunately, oftentimes they're not. Don't be fooled by the clever packaging – bottled juices and smoothies can be high in sugar, so always read the label. Make your own fresh fruit juices and smoothies from scratch instead.

MYTH: LOW FAT, NO FAT, ZERO CALORIES, NATURAL AND SUGAR FREE MEANS IT'S GOOD FOR YOU, RIGHT?

Unless you've made the food yourself at home, it can be hard to say what chemicals, preservatives, additives, trans fats and sugars have been used, to name just a few. Manufacturers have no obligation to help you to be healthy or to even be 100% sincere about their product. They use clever marketing to drive sales, even if that means pulling the wool over their customers' eyes. Terms like *homemade* and *natural* actually have no legal meaning whatsoever and offer no indication of the nutritional value of the product. Terms like *low fat* or *no added sugar* don't necessarily mean the food is healthier either. Rather than buy products based on their label or their promises, **opt for simple, nutritious food that hasn't changed much as a result of processing**.

MYTH: ALL FRUIT AND VEGETABLES ARE CREATED EQUAL

Fruit and vegetables are both important and they are both super healthy, offering a wide range of vitamins, minerals and antioxidants. But all fruit and veg offer different nutrients. Some are high in natural carbs and others are high in natural sugars, which needs to be accounted for. Fruit contains a lot of natural sugars, as do vegetables like carrots and peas. Also, natural carbohydrates like white potatoes are high in starch.

Of course, all fruit and vegetables are healthy and should be included in your diet, but you should eat more vegetables than fruit. **Aim to include vegetables in almost every meal and fruit in smaller portions.** Fruit is also a great healthy treat that has way more health benefits than any junk food.

MYTH: YOUR METABOLISM SLOWS DOWN WITH AGE, CAUSING WEIGHT GAIN

We naturally lose muscle as we age. A woman in her 60s won't have the same ability to grow and maintain muscle as a 25-year-old woman, but genuine changes in metabolism are actually microscopic. **The real reason people tend to gain weight with age is as a result of lifestyle changes and the reduction of muscle, which means a natural gain in body fat.** Your metabolism stays fairly stable throughout your life. In their book *Biomarkers*, researchers W. Evans and I.H. Rosenberg state that you can prevent muscle loss by maintaining a healthy diet and continuing to lift weights.

MYTH: YOU'RE NOT GETTING RESULTS BECAUSE OF YOUR GENETICS

You may have an inherent disposition to put on weight or you may be the opposite and have a hard time gaining weight, but that doesn't mean you can't make significant improvements and maintain them. **Blaming your genetics as the reason you're not getting results is a total cop-out.** Two girls may sport the exact same dress size but look totally different. Maybe one has longer legs and the other has a bigger bum. These two girls may follow the exact same diet plan and workout regime and give the exact same effort but get totally different (but still positive) results. Just because it might take you longer to build up a booty or drop body fat in your stomach area doesn't mean you can't get there. It just might take a little longer than the person you're comparing yourself to.

So quit using your genes as an excuse, because hard work and dedication along with the right diet and workout plans works. Avoid overeating or undereating; read more about your basal metabolic rate on page 148, and you'll have no excuses.

MYTH: IT'S NOT YOUR FAULT IF YOU'RE NOT MAKING PROGRESS

You can blame everyone and everything under the sun for the lack of success you're having or for the reason you aren't improving, but the only person responsible is the one you see in the mirror. Sometimes you just need to stand up and take ownership of your actions. Maybe you're not being honest with yourself or maybe you're not aware of your actions. You can continue the way you're going, but then you risk staying the same: being stuck at your personal average when you have every possibility of being your absolute best. The only person who can change your life is you, so the people you blame can't help you – they're busy working on their own lives. Everybody has the ability to do anything they put their mind to. **You are not destined to stay the same – *you* decide how your life will turn out.**

MYTH: HEALTHY EATING IS EXPENSIVE

There is a big misconception out there that eating healthy is more expensive than eating junk food, but I simply don't believe it's true. I have put this into practice myself, so I know that it is 100% possible to eat clean on a budget. Your budget is a very individual thing, of course, but if you're determined to eat healthy, you will make it work.

Sure, you can buy a fast food burger for one euro, but you can also buy a chicken breast or a head of broccoli for that price. But when you start to weigh up the differences, you'll quickly realise that the good food is way more valuable because of its nutritive value. **Instead of asking why healthy food is more expensive, have you ever stopped to think about why junk food is so cheap?** It might seem like you're getting good value in terms of your wallet, but you certainly won't be getting good value in terms of your body and your health – it can be a case of paying the grocer, not the doctor.

GROCERY SHOP FOR SUCCESS

Don't simply presume that you will eat healthy – you need to be prepared and proactive about your food choices and schedule. If you are prepared, organised and efficient, you will have much greater success. If you're not well prepared, you'll only be putting yourself in a position to cheat on your plan. You'll be surprised at how easily it becomes second nature once you've been doing it for a while and when you start seeing the results.

The diet plans in Chapter 8 don't mean you'll be chained to the kitchen and your life won't have to revolve around it. The plans are there to give guidelines, support and motivation and to make eating healthy that much easier. Being organised can also stop you from making bad choices and it encourages you to stay on the right path. Make things easy and convenient for yourself, because something that is difficult will be harder to maintain.

Meal prep doesn't just mean lunch boxes and cold food. It's about the process in which you manage and control your food for the week. It boils down to thinking ahead and preparing to be successful. **They say 'if you fail to prepare, then prepare to fail', and that is certainly true when it comes to planning your meals.**

MEAL PREP STARTS WITH YOUR DIET PLAN

Make sure you know exactly what's in your weekly diet plan so that you can make a precise grocery list for all seven days, including breakfasts, lunches, dinners and snacks. Routine is fundamental to the success of this process, so pick a day that suits you to go shopping as well as the day or time that suits you to get everything ready. I like to shop on a Sunday so that I'm all set for another successful week of eating great food for my body – plus nothing beats being organised for the Monday.

When you shop, stick to your plan, your list and your budget. Don't throw random things into your basket just for the sake of it – avoid buying sweet treats and junk food, because if it's in your house, you will eat it. When you're having a cheat meal or having a treat, buy it that day. Never keep junk food lying around, because you're only fooling yourself. **Don't put yourself into a situation where you're only setting yourself up to fail with your food.**

Getting your food ready for the week could mean cooking it now and freezing some food for later in the week or chopping vegetables ahead of time. Find a roll-out rhythm and routine that suits your lifestyle. And be sure to invest in some good-quality lunch boxes that are BPA free and microwavable – they're a seriously good investment.

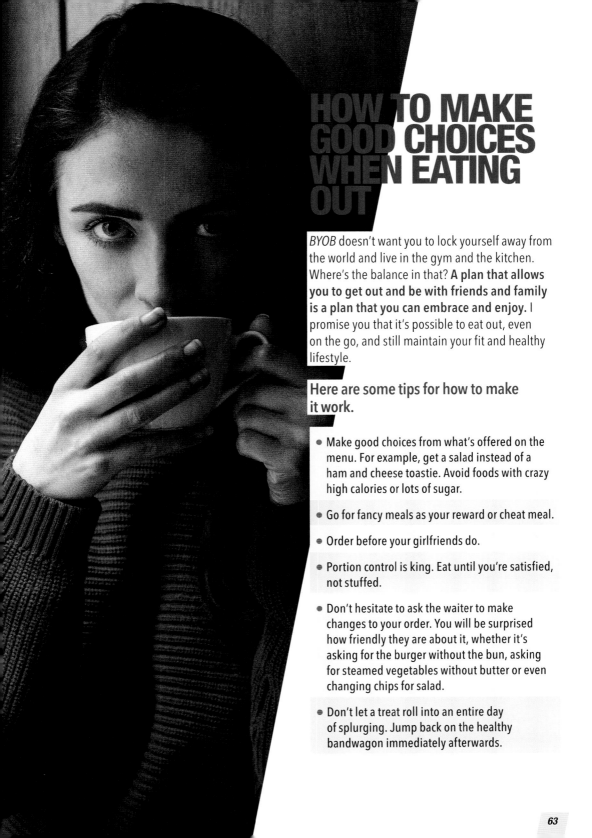

HOW TO MAKE GOOD CHOICES WHEN EATING OUT

BYOB doesn't want you to lock yourself away from the world and live in the gym and the kitchen. Where's the balance in that? **A plan that allows you to get out and be with friends and family is a plan that you can embrace and enjoy.** I promise you that it's possible to eat out, even on the go, and still maintain your fit and healthy lifestyle.

Here are some tips for how to make it work.

- Make good choices from what's offered on the menu. For example, get a salad instead of a ham and cheese toastie. Avoid foods with crazy high calories or lots of sugar.

- Go for fancy meals as your reward or cheat meal.

- Order before your girlfriends do.

- Portion control is king. Eat until you're satisfied, not stuffed.

- Don't hesitate to ask the waiter to make changes to your order. You will be surprised how friendly they are about it, whether it's asking for the burger without the bun, asking for steamed vegetables without butter or even changing chips for salad.

- Don't let a treat roll into an entire day of splurging. Jump back on the healthy bandwagon immediately afterwards.

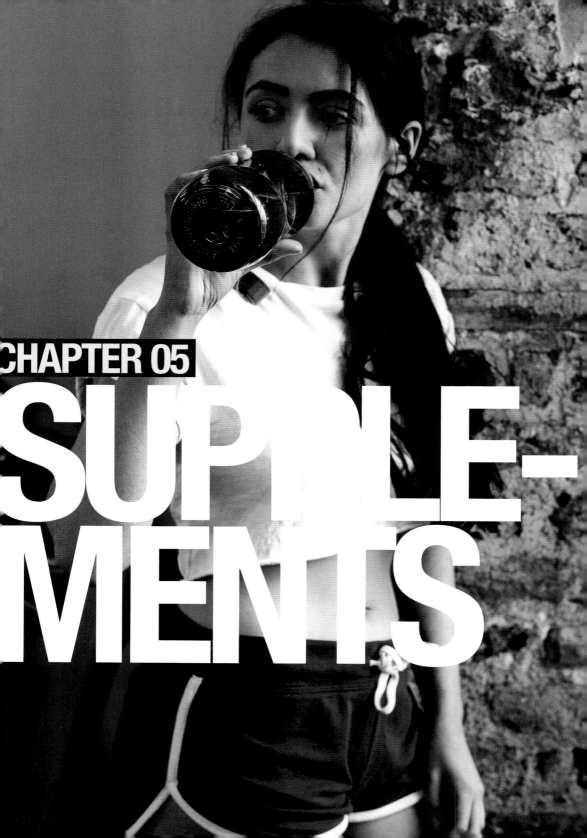

CHAPTER 05

SUPPLE-
MENTS

Let's be honest: most people don't take in enough vitamins and minerals through their diet. Ideally we should meet all our daily nutrition needs through wholesome, nutritious food, but we don't. That's where supplements come in.

A dietary supplement is intended to add extra nutritional value to the diet. Supplements can be a convenient and handy way to improve, but you should never use them as a replacement for food. Think of them as an add-on that can be used to aid your recovery, growth, weight loss and overall health. Supplements can't do it alone, but when used with a good nutrition and exercise plan, you can really capitalise on the benefits. The whole idea is to maximise your efforts and get the most out of the work you're doing.

WHY TAKE SUPPLEMENTS?

Supplements aren't just for men and beefheads – women can get as much benefit from supplements as men can. You can increase your results and improve your health, growth and recovery. A lot of people feel uncomfortable visiting their local sports nutrition shop, but that large man behind the counter is probably hugely knowledgeable and will help you pick the perfect products for your needs. Alternatively, you can shop online or visit your local health food store, which will have just as many products and the staff will have just as much knowledge.

Supplements aren't miracle pills, but they can give you a helping hand. Sometimes a strong supplement plan can be as simple as taking a daily multivitamin and multimineral. Or depending on your goals, you can use dietary supplements to help you get the most out of your recovery and thus aid growth. Not only will they help you get the most out of your new plan, but the Council for Responsible Nutrition says they will also help fight off unwanted colds and flu and will have a positive impact on your skin, hair and energy. Supplements are also essential in fighting chronic illness as a result of poor nutrition.

But just like every other aspect of the *BYOB* plan, supplements will only work if you do and if you know how to use them. They are meant to improve your health, not diminish it, but you have to use them in a responsible, informed way. As the pie chart shows, a successful fitness life is all about balance, and supplements have a part to play in that.

This pie chart is a breakdown of my own fitness wheel. As you can see, it doesn't include social life, work life or sleep, just the basics. If you can include all these elements and devote the right amount of time and effort to each, you will have great success with your goals and results.

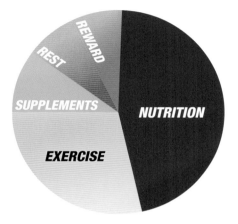

HOW TO GET STARTED WITH SUPPLEMENTS

The great thing about supplements is that they are so easy to take. I typically do it in the morning and now it's second nature.

The best way to start with a supplements stack is to keep it simple, then progress as your knowledge and understanding develop. Start by taking a daily multivitamin/multimineral and some vitamin C and try a protein shake after your workout. These three things will get you on the right track to becoming a supplements wizard. Don't go overboard buying expensive products that will just sit on the shelf, and

be sure to take the recommended amount at the right time – anything more than that is just a waste.

SUPPLEMENT MYTHS

MYTH: ALL SUPPLEMENTS ARE THE SAME

There is a huge difference in the quality of supplements, and the NHS in the UK warns against taking low-quality products. Again, instead of asking why some products are so expensive, ask yourself why the cheap products are so *in*expensive. Look for good-quality, highly recommended brands and don't be afraid to compare labels. Avoid supplements with fillers and unnecessary toxic chemicals.

MYTH: DRINKING PROTEIN SHAKES WILL MAKE YOU BULKY OR FAT

Protein is essential for the maintenance and growth of healthy lean muscle tissue. The only way to get bulky or to gain body fat is by overeating.

MYTH: SUPPLEMENTS ARE STEROIDS AND ARE BAD FOR YOUR KIDNEYS

This is a major misconception about supplements like creatine and glutamine. The truth is that they are the exact same as the vitamins and minerals you take on a daily basis, just with different functions and benefits. Creatine helps your muscles to get the nutrients they need to perform and grow, while glutamine minimises muscle breakdown and supports protein metabolism.

MYTH: SUPPLEMENTS ALONE WILL MAKE ME SHREDDED

Sorry, but there is no magic pill except hard work. Yes, supplements alone can improve your health and sleep, reduce stress and boost your immune system, but they cannot make you shredded or make you gain muscle and strength. Utilising them with your training is what will help you get shredded and toned.

MYTH: FAT BURNERS ARE DANGEROUS

False. Fat burners are a great addition to a weight loss programme. When used in a safe way they can help to increase your metabolism and help your body to burn some extra fat. However, due to its high caffeine content, this product should not be abused or taken in the wrong way. As you know, the most effective way to burn fat is through diet, and that is 80% of the battle. Fat burners can act as a little boost, especially with energy.

FUNCTIONS AND BENEFITS OF SUPPLEMENTS

MULTIVITAMINS

What does it do? Multivitamins help to maintain or improve overall health when taken as an add-on to a healthy diet in order to guarantee you take in enough nutrients every day. For convenience, take a multivitamin/multimineral combo.

What are the benefits? Multivitamins help you to convert food into energy, boost your immune system and support overall function and health, from your bones to your skin to your digestive system.

When do I take it? Any time during the day is suitable, but getting into a routine with supplements will mean greater success. I recommend taking a multivitamin in the morning with breakfast.

How much do I take? Typically you take two tablets once a day, but read the label for directions as brands may vary.

MULTIMINERALS

What does it do? Like multivitamins, multiminerals help maintain normal bodily functions and support a healthy diet. A multimineral supplement ensures you get your required mineral intake per day. For convenience, take a multivitamin/multimineral combo.

What are the benefits? Multiminerals maintain healthy liver and kidney function, promote eye health and hearth health, transport oxygen and assist in energy production.

When do I take it? Any time during the day, along with the rest of your supplements. I recommend taking it in the morning with breakfast.

How much do I take? Typically you take two tablets once a day, but read the label for directions as brands may vary.

WHEY PROTEIN CONCENTRATE

What does it do? Whey protein powder is derived from milk and is high in protein. It is the fastest-digesting protein that you can take.

What are the benefits? Taking whey protein stimulates muscle growth through protein synthesis and aids blood flow to the muscles, which helps in recovery. It's also a great way to meet the protein requirements in your daily diet plan.

When do I take it? The best time to take a protein shake is post-workout, usually no later than 20–30 minutes after a gym session for maximum benefits. Protein shakes are also super handy for anyone who hasn't got time to make a meal and needs a quick fix. This is not a meal replacement, though – it's just handy for those times when you're stuck.

How much do I take? Typically one scoop after a workout.

WHEY PROTEIN ISOLATE

What does it do? Whey protein isolate is similar to whey protein concentrate, as they are both derived from milk. Whey protein isolate is more processed but offers more protein per unit than whey.

What are the benefits? Whey protein isolate offers the same benefits as whey concentrate. However, it's lower in carbs and calories, and because it's more processed it can lack the nutrients that are in the concentrate.

When do I take it? For optimal results, have one shake 20–30 minutes post-workout.

How much do I take? One scoop.

PRE-WORKOUT

What does it do? Pre-workout is a sports supplement that increases performance. As the name suggestions, you take it prior to a workout. Pre-workout is not an essential component of a supplement stack, but some people use it for an added boost during workouts.

What are the benefits? The biggest benefit of pre-workout is an increase in energy, intensity and focus during a workout. It also offers muscle-developing and stamina- and strength-increasing properties.

When do I take it? 30–40 minutes before a workout.

How much do I take? One serving before a workout. See the instructions for the recommended dose.

FAT BURNERS

What does it do? Fat burner tablets, or thermogenics, assist in fat loss by boosting metabolism. The main ingredient is caffeine, which is one of the most effective weight loss chemicals according to research by M.S. Westerterp-Plantenga, M.P. Lejeune and E.M. Kovacs. published in the *Obesity Research* journal. Because it's a stimulant, you should only take small quantities to support your efforts in the gym and your healthy eating plan. Fat burners are not a miracle diet pill and using them on their own won't help you reach your fitness goals.

What are the benefits? More energy and an improved metabolism, which results in fat loss.

When do I take it? Due to its caffeine content, you should take them early in the day - with breakfast is a perfect time.

How much do I take? This totally depends on your tolerance level, but start with one per day, with the potential to increase to two tablets a day. Again, follow the instructions on the label and never take more than the recommended dose.

CASEIN

What does it do? Casein is a form of protein powder. It's a slow-releasing protein source that supplies nutrients and amino acids to the muscle over the entire day.

What are the benefits? Casein offers muscle support and fuel over a long period of time.

When do I take it? Casein should be taken in the evening, even before bedtime, to take advantage of the slow-releasing protein source that will support your muscles while you sleep.

How much do I take? One scoop.

FISH OILS

What does it do? Fish oils are essential for maintaining health and for reducing inflammation.

What are the benefits? Fish oils maintain a healthy cholesterol level and bone health and reduce inflammation.

When do I take it? Take with the rest of your supplements in the morning.

How much do I take? Typically two tablets, but read the label to check your particular brand.

BRANCH CHAIN AMINO ACIDS (BCAAs)

What does it do? BCAAs are a supplement that supports muscles.

What are the benefits? It improves exercise and weight-training performance and reduces muscle breakdown.

When do I take it? The best times to use BCAAs are before, during or after a workout.

How much do I take? It depends on whether you're using a tablet or powder, but it's usually two tablets or one scoop of powder. Follow the directions on the label.

CREATINE

What does it do? It supports muscle growth, repair and performance.

What are the benefits? It increases blood flow to the muscles, which promotes cell growth.

When do I take it? The best time is after a workout, but it's also beneficial in the morning or before a workout.

How much do I take? 5g

CONJUGATED LINOLEIC ACID (CLA)

What does it do? CLA is a support for lean muscle. It also acts as a fat burner and even has anti-cancer properties.

What are the benefits? It increases your metabolic rate and fat-burning mechanism, supports muscle growth, aids immunity and lowers cholesterol.

When do I take it? You can take it at any time, but it's convenient to take it in the morning with breakfast.

How much do I take? Your intake will depend on whether you are using it for muscle support or fat loss. For fat loss, you should take roughly 3,000mg a day.

L-GLUTAMINE

What does it do? Glutamine is an amino acid found in the body. It is the most common amino acid in your muscles.

What are the benefits? It assists muscle growth, repair and recovery and supports healthy brain function.

When do I take it? After a workout for maximum benefit or in the morning.

How much do I take? One serving, as per your brand's suggestions.

VITAMIN B COMPLEX

What does it do? Vitamin B complex includes eight different B vitamins that are water soluble.

What are the benefits? Vitamin B is essential for normal bodily function, as it helps transport nutrients around the body, turning food into energy, and it assists in the production of red blood cells.

When do I take it? In the morning along with the rest of your supplements.

How much do I take? Always make sure to take 100% of your daily intake. Follow the instructions on the label of your particular brand, as it could be two tablets or one capsule.

VITAMIN C

What does it do? Vitamin C is a water-soluble vitamin. It's also called ascorbic acid.

What are the benefits? Vitamin C is important for maintaining and developing connective tissue in the body. It's also a strong antioxidant that can relieve the symptoms and reduce the length of the common cold. It also increases absorption of iron.

When do I take it? In the morning along with the rest of your supplements.

How much do I take? Always make sure to take 100% of your daily intake. Follow the instructions on the label of your particular brand, as it could be two tablets or one capsule.

VITAMIN D

What does it do? Helps absorb calcium into the body.

What are the benefits? Maintains healthy body function and bones.

When do I take it? In the morning along with the rest of your supplements.

How much do I take? Always make sure to take 100% of your daily intake. Follow the instructions on the label of your particular brand, as it could be two tablets or one capsule.

(Sources: *American Journal of Clinical Nutrition,* American Society for Nutrition, *Dietary Reference Intakes: The Essential Guide to Nutrient Requirements, European Journal of Applied Physiology,* Examine.com, Harvard Health Publications, Harvard Medical School 'Listing of vitamins', International Society of Sports Nutrition Symposium, *Journal of Nutrition, Journal of Obesity, Journal of Sports Medicine and Doping Studies, Journal of the International Society of Sports Nutrition, Merriam-Webster Dictionary, Molecular and Cellular Biochemistry,* National Strength and Conditioning Association, *Nutrition Journal, Sports Medicine,* University of Rochester Medical Center Health Encyclopedia, US National Library of Medicine Medical Encyclopedia and www.bodybuilding.com.)

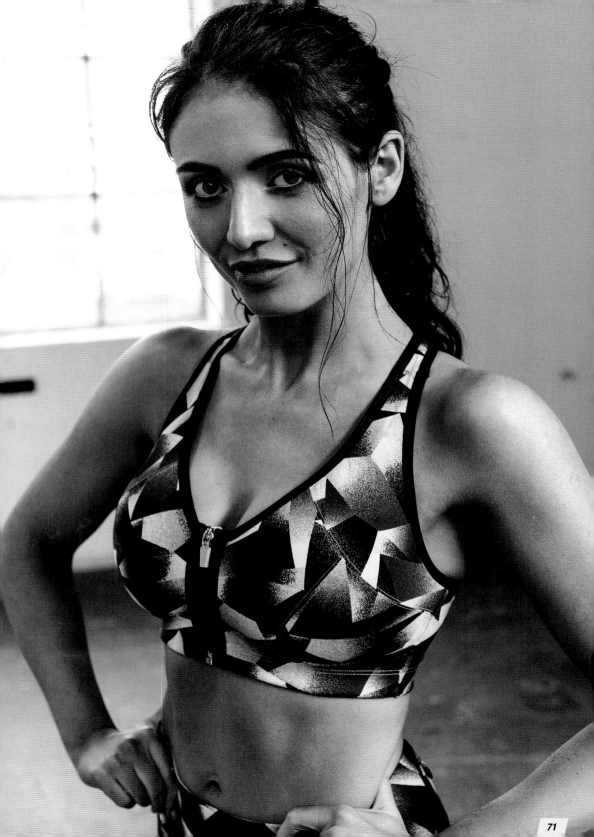

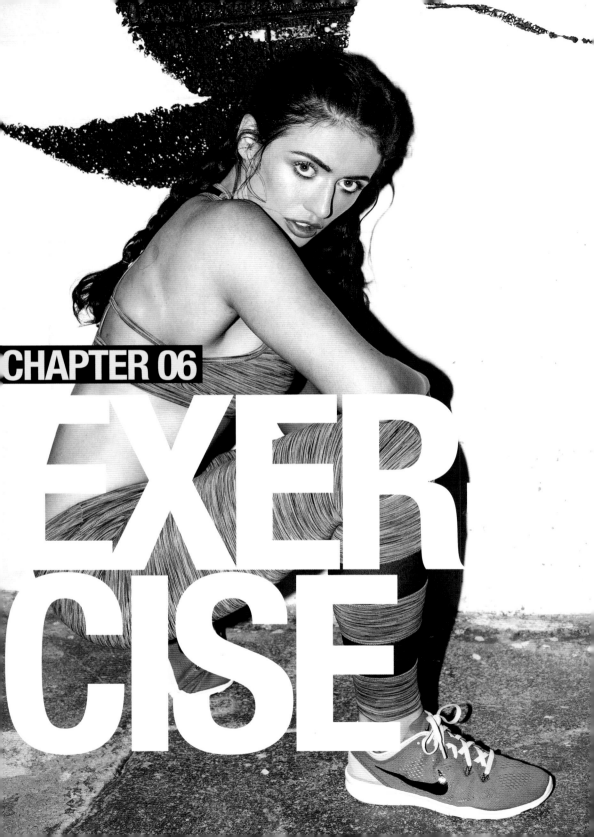

CHAPTER 06

EXER CISE

This is my favourite part of the entire book because exercise is the fun part! This chapter will build your knowledge and your confidence by briefly explaining what happens when you exercise. I'll also list some of the essentials that will help you to get started, debunk some myths, outline the differences between strength training and cardio as well as the two types of weightlifting movements, tell you why warming up and good technique are vital, and encourage you to turn your weaknesses into a strength.

EXERCISE IS WHAT CAUSES REAL CHANGE

It can take quite some time to get your head around a healthy diet and master it, but **exercise offers an immediate sense of achievement**. This was the major reason for the turnaround in my life. Yes, transforming my body was an amazing extra and taking part in bodybuilding shows gave me back a sense of purpose, but from day one, exercise gave me a euphoric sense of happiness, empowerment and self-confidence.

Before my fitness epiphany I enjoyed sports and being outdoorsy, but the truth is that any time I tried to do the gym thing, I hated it. I dreaded a workout and I hated the effort and the pain, but now I love it, from throwing on my comfy sweat bottoms and baggy T-shirt to packing my gym bag with all the supplements I need for intra- and post-workout gains, jumping in my car and turning the music on full blast to get myself pumped for my upcoming session, arriving at the gym and saying my hellos, then sticking on my headphones and boom, time to hammer my workout.

For me, exercise is now a daily ritual, almost like going to mass except I'm paying my respects to the heavy weights I'm about to smash and the mental challenges I'm going to overcome in the space of a one-hour workout. All right, so that all sounds pretty intense and emotional, and if you don't feel like that about a workout, don't worry, that's okay! The most important thing is that you don't hate working out. It may take a while to get to that point, but stay strong until then. The time will come when you start to see results from your efforts, whether it's a growth in muscle, a more defined stomach, a reduction in cellulite or even an increase in strength. That will be an extra incentive to drive you and to push you to keep going, but until that happens, just suck it up, roll your sleeves up and do the hard work.

"LEARN TO LOVE THE BURN!"

Exercise facilitates body change. As you learned in the previous chapters, food will fuel you and help you lose body fat and supplements will give you a helping hand too, but **exercise is what causes real change**. If you have always wanted to be toned and have a full, perky bum, the only way to do it is to lift weights, and to lift properly. I was very lucky to have the support of an amazing coach who taught me the importance of lifting with proper technique rather than just going through the motions. Accurate training can drastically change your body in ways you never could have imagined. This chapter is going to give you the tools to do just that.

BE SMART ABOUT YOUR BODY

The key to making the most of your workouts is knowledge – and why wouldn't you want to maximise your gym sessions? Yet the truth is that most women aren't training the right way or using smart technique, meaning they are essentially only seeing minimal results. I also see it very often in women who are overtraining. **Be smart about exercise by using your brain, not just your body.**

Have you ever got stuck in a gym regime and wondered why you weren't getting results? Do you know what body part you're working or what the reason is for doing a particular exercise? Are you engaging the muscle correctly? Are you looking after your joints and your back? There's a lot more to this than just going to the gym and swinging weights around the place aimlessly.

By training with knowledge, you can see massive changes for your efforts. Mastering information is the key to success, but exercise is easy to understand. By being smart about your body, like understanding what happens during exercise and knowing more about the body part you're training, you can get more out of your exercise regime.

WHAT IS EXERCISE?

Exercise means taking part in physical activity with the goal of maintaining or improving health. People take on physical activity for recreational reasons, to lose weight, to gain muscle or for a range of other reasons. Exercise can be tailored to your individual needs and goals and it can literally transform your existing body and its capabilities. **Everybody has the ability to improve using exercise, whether it's physically, mentally or even both.** Exercise is a fundamental part of life, and anyone who wants to live a long and healthy life should exercise regularly, ideally every day. The WHO, Mayo Clinic, American Heart Association and the Office of Disease Prevention and Health Promotion as well as Get Active Ireland all recommend exercising at least three times a week or 30 minutes a day, but if you're looking for significant improvements, you should aim to be physical five or six times a week.

There is no one style of fitness that suits everyone, and the same applies to physical activity. My opinion is that whatever your fitness calling may be, make sure you have a good balance between strength training and cardiovascular activity. The main goal is to improve performance, improve your body and maintain a healthy heart.

WHAT ARE THE BENEFITS OF EXERCISE?

- Fights illness and disease
- Increases bone density
- Controls body weight
- Boosts energy
- Fights depression
- Helps maintain a healthy mind
- Improves your confidence and self-esteem
- Improves your complexion and hair
- Develops more muscle and muscle definition
- Improves heart and brain health
- Helps to burn body fat
- It's a social activity
- Improves sleep
- Increases sexual function

WHAT HAPPENS TO YOUR BODY WHEN YOU EXERCISE?

Exercise is a *positive* stress on the body, unlike the mental stresses we inflict on ourselves through work, relationships, our social lives and emotions. Exercise offers huge health and body benefits, both inside and out. Doing physical activity on a regular basis has rewards for your entire body: your muscles, brain, lungs, heart, ligaments and tendons all benefit. By now you know the benefits of exercise, from controlling weight to maintaining good health and fighting disease, but do you really know what's going on underneath your skin? You can of course enjoy a successful active life without knowing all the ins and outs, but you should at least have a basic understanding of what's going on. Remember, knowledge is power, and the more you know about your body, the better. Plus I bet you'll be amazed at how everything is connected, from your breathing to your results.

When you start exercising your muscles need oxygen, so at this stage you will no doubt notice that your breathing is getting heavier and your breaths are much bigger. The increase in your breathing increases your heart rate, which in turn increases the blood flow around your body. Have you ever heard anyone at the gym or online talking about being 'pumped'? Well, that's exactly what it's referring to: when your blood vessels dilate to allow more oxygen into them. It's the same reason why we get an embarrassingly red face during a workout, so embrace it if it happens because it means your body is working. Have you ever noticed that a workout gets easier as the weeks go by and you see improvements in both your capabilities and intensity? It means your muscles are using oxygen more efficiently, which is what lowers your heart rate.

WHAT HAPPENS TO YOUR MUSCLES WHEN YOU EXERCISE?

When exercising, your muscles need energy to move and function, so your body utilises stored glucose (glycogen), which comes from the food you have eaten. It also uses adenosine triphosphate (ATP). After all the glucose and ATP stores have been used up, your body calls on oxygen to facilitate even more ATP.

Lifting weights causes tiny tears within the muscle fibres, and when these tears heal they become larger and stronger. **It is in the healing that your muscles grow, hence the importance of eating to repair and rest.** If you overtrain and continuously tear muscle fibres, they begin to deteriorate, which is why it's important to prioritise recovery.

WHAT HAPPENS TO YOUR HEART WHEN YOU EXERCISE?

Exercising increases the heart rate, which in turn circulates more oxygen around your body. This increase then transports oxygenated blood to the muscles, which you need to perform. **The more you exercise, the better your heart gets at this process**, which means you will perform better. In addition, new blood vessels are produced during exercise, resulting in lower blood pressure.

WHAT HAPPENS TO YOUR BRAIN WHEN YOU EXERCISE?

Firstly, your brain produces glutamate and dopamine to get your body moving, allowing you to actually do the exercise or activity at hand.

As we've already discussed, the major impact of exercise is an increase in blood around your body. **This also positively**

affects your brain, which makes it function at a higher level both during exercise and afterwards. What's more, the NHS, Mayo Clinic, Harvard Medical School and Alzheimer's Association state that the increased blood flow to the brain can fight diseases like Alzheimer's and reduce the chance of having a stoke. Plus you also already know that the mental benefits of exercise are due to the increase in serotonin, which is responsible for a happy mind.

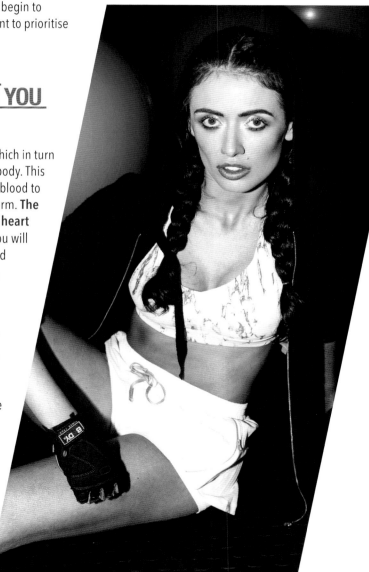

In addition to all of these, exercise also boosts lung, joint and bone health.

WHAT HAPPENS WHEN YOU DON'T EXERCISE?

Have you ever heard the saying 'either make time for fitness or make time for illness'? It really says it all. **If you don't make time for good nutrition and your mental and physical health today, then you will no doubt suffer the consequences later in life.** A lot of people think that just because they are naturally slim that it automatically makes them fit and healthy, while others think being fit is a luxury, not a necessity.

So what are the real dangers of living an inactive, lazy life? Here are a few of them, according to the WHO and NHS, amongst others:

- Increased risk of cancer
- Higher chance of diabetes
- Higher chance of chronic illness
- Depression
- Irregular mood
- Unmanageable stress levels
- Higher chance of being overweight
- Higher chance of being unhappy with your weight
- Unable to maintain weight
- More likely to get injured due to weaker joints and bones
- Less muscle, meaning more loose skin
- Higher blood pressure

HOW LONG DOES IT TAKE IT TO SEE RESULTS FROM EXERCISE?

Everybody wants quick results, but Rome wasn't built in a day, and neither can the body of your dreams. You are going to see immediate results in terms of your nutrition, including more energy, more focus and improved mood, but how long will it really take to see the results of your efforts when it comes to exercising?

Firstly, I want to highlight again the importance of having realistic goals and being patient with making slow but steady progress. By doing this, you can maintain your results in the long term and avoid falling off the bandwagon.

It is possible to see significant changes in your body after as little as eight weeks, but don't try to fast track that. It might take you a year or even two years to reach your ultimate ideal goal, but remember, this is a lifestyle and one that you want to maintain forever. Don't look for a quick fix. Buckle down, work hard and set realistic goals, like losing one pound a month. You will see an impressive increase in muscle in as little as six months if you stay consistent and do the right training. **Don't look for shortcuts, because the changes will happen.** Wait and see.

EXERCISE ESSENTIALS

Now that you know some of the benefits of exercise, here are some basics to get you going. Of course, many of these items are in no way essential or fundamental to your success – you don't have to spend any extra money to achieve your fitness goals. These are just some nice items that make life that little bit easier or are recommended if you're ready to take things up a notch.

COMFORTABLE GYM CLOTHES

This is a very individual thing, and like all aspects of this lifestyle, being individual is key. Some people love wearing the latest trends and putting on their favourite Nike crop top, while others prefer to work out in an extra large men's T-shirt. There is no uniform in a fitness club or if you're hitting the pavement for a run, so pick what works for you. **The most important thing is that you feel 100% comfortable in what you are wearing.** Wear something that isn't going to annoy you or distract you during a workout session. It might seem like an obvious point to make, but people feel pressured to wear the latest trends and spend a lot of money on sportswear. I can promise you now that nobody else cares what you have on in the gym, so don't waste your time thinking you need to dress up for the benefit of other people. They're too busy doing their workout. So remember, the key considerations are clothes that are comfortable, suit your body shape and give you freedom of movement.

A GOOD SPORTS BRA

I have seen some horrific scenes of the wrong bra mixed with an intense workout, and it is not pretty. When you go to the gym you should be prepared and comfortable. Your workout should be the main priority above all else without the distraction of unruly breasts. Plus **not wearing the appropriate sports bra can have some serious consequences**, not least of which is saggy breasts. When women don't support their breasts they risk damaging ligaments called Cooper's ligaments, and when these are damaged they can never be repaired. Damaged Cooper's ligaments cause breasts to hang or sag. Of course, the more obvious reasons for wearing the right sports bra include being comfortable and preventing pain, so invest in a good one and put it to use.

PROPERLY LACED TRAINERS

At the risk of sounding like a PE teacher, **lacing your trainers properly is essential**. Shoes have laces for a reason, not for decorative purposes. If you want to get the most out of your workout, then supporting your feet, ankles and joints is fundamental. Remember, you're at the gym to get results, not to look cool, so lace up and don't run the risk of an unnecessary injury.

A GOOD GYM BAG

Another obvious one, but **having a great gym bag that you can use every day is a solid part of your routine**. I keep it handy and visible, which encourages me to go. I always keep my essentials in there, like my water bottle, intra- and post-workout supplements and shower products, and then I pack the rest of my items as needed. Also, make sure your bag is big enough to make things more convenient for yourself.

A LARGE WATER BOTTLE – THE BIGGER, THE BETTER

We are not messing around here. It's time to get results – big results – so bringing a tiny bottle of water to the gym is pointless. **Invest in a large bottle**, which will encourage you to drink more. Try to bring a bottle that holds 2 litres of water or more and keep it in your gym bag.

INTRA- AND POST-WORKOUT SUPPLEMENTS

If you don't bring them, then you aren't going to take them. Always keep them in your gym bag, separate from your morning supplements. Whether it's your protein powder, creatine, glutamine or BCAAs, make sure they're in your bag.

SHAKER

I like to have a couple of shakers around the place. They have a short lifespan, but they are reasonably cheap. **Keep one at home and another one in your gym bag**, because how else can you have your post-workout shake and supplements? Always make sure to rinse your shaker immediately after you finish your shake.

TOWEL

Carrying a gym towel is good exercise etiquette. It means you respect your environment, your equipment and the people around you. Leaving a machine sweaty is just rude, so be a good sport and always carry a towel to wipe things down.

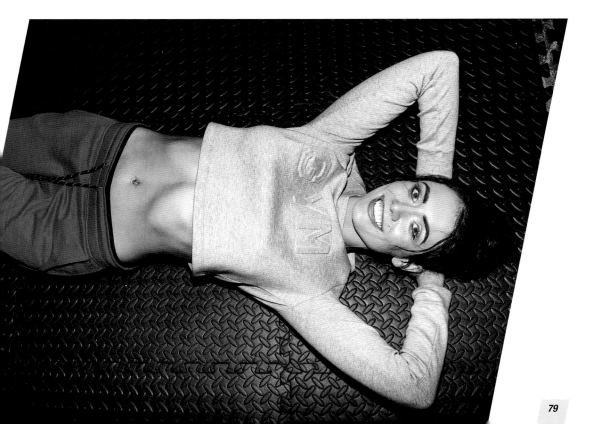

HEADPHONES AND A GREAT PLAYLIST

Some people don't need music for motivation, but I am not one of those people. Plus sometimes the tunes on offer in your local leisure club are not up to par, so **have your favourite songs ready to go**. It's a great way to get inspired and to have fun during a workout.

RESISTANCE BANDS AND CABLE

These are not essential and there is more than enough equipment in your gym to do all of your workouts. I just love these and think **every fitness queen should have them**. They are great to have at home if you want to do a workout, if you're travelling or on holidays. They are also a great way to warm up before a big workout and engage the muscle to wake it up.

AB WHEEL

Again, this is not an essential piece of equipment, since you can find them sometimes in your local gym, but they are really affordable and are a handy piece of equipment to have at home for a killer ab workout.

SKIPPING ROPE

Another great addition to your home equipment. Skipping is so much fun and it's a great way to do some cardio at home or outside.

MEAL PREP BAG

I think these are super. They make life so much easier if you're the type of person who really takes organisation seriously.

WEIGHTLIFTING GLOVES

I like to wear these when I'm lifting big and doing movements like deadlifts. You could also try weightlifting chalk. Both are used for improving grip and can also help you avoid getting hard calluses on your hands as a result of lifting weights.

WEIGHTLIFTING BELT

A lot of women look at the typical man in the gym wearing a belt and feel totally intimidated, but a weightlifting belt offers back support and reduces strain on the spine during heavy lifting. Something to think about as your confidence – and the amount of weight you're lifting – increases.

KNEE OR JOINT SUPPORT

If you have any previous injuries or feel that something is weak, it's important to be responsible and safe and support it. There is no point in adding extra strain on something that is weakened, as you're only sure to injure it further. As always, you should get advice from your GP before starting any fitness programme..

A WORKOUT PLAN OR DIARY

Lastly, **you need a plan**, whether it's your gym programme card or a little diary that you can carry with you, because without it you are arriving to the gym unprepared. And remember, if you fail to prepare, then prepare to fail. Make life that much easier for yourself and come to the gym ready, already knowing what your full workout for the day consists of. After a while, your exercise plan will become second nature and you won't need a piece of paper to lead your workout.

EXERCISE, WEIGHTLIFTING AND MUSCLE MYTHS

MYTH: MUSCLE TURNS TO FAT WHEN YOU STOP EXERCISING

This is simply impossible. Fat and muscle are two totally separate entities, so no, **muscle can never turn to body fat**. In fact, when you stop exercising your muscles get smaller, and unless you reduce your calorie intake appropriately, you will gain size as a result of body fat.

MYTH: LIFTING WEIGHTS WILL MAKE YOU BULKY

I hear this one all the time, from *I don't want to lift weights because I don't want to look like Arnold Schwarzenegger* or *Oh Kelly, don't get any bigger.* The truth is that **lifting weights improves overall proportions** – for example, it makes your waist look smaller. But it's a myth that just won't die when it comes to women lifting weights. When women get significantly larger due to weightlifting, it's because they want to. It involves years of intense and precise weightlifting along with eating a seriously large number of calories. For the average woman who lifts weights, it's almost impossible to get bulky. I assure you that eating junk food or a party lifestyle will give you a bulky physique, but not weight training. Women don't have the testosterone or hormones to get large; we are simply not designed like that. I read a great fitness quote recently: 'Lifting weights won't make you a giant bodybuilder, just like going for a jog won't make you an Olympic athlete.' So don't be afraid to lift heavy. Lifting weights will make things perkier, curvier and give you your dream silhouette.

> ## "LIFTING WEIGHTS WON'T MAKE YOU BULKY – TOO MANY CUPCAKES WILL."

MYTH: CRUNCHES CREATE SIX PACKS

Doing crunches actually burns very few calories in comparison to other activities. If you're wondering why you can't see your six pack or even a toned, tight stomach despite doing endless sit-ups, it's because it's hidden behind a layer of body fat. **So don't rely solely on crunches.** Maintaining a healthy diet and doing cardiovascular activity and more intense core work will help you see those abs in no time.

MYTH: LIFTING WEIGHTS IS DANGEROUS

The only activity that is truly dangerous is inactivity. Your body wants you to exercise and move. It's possible to injure yourself every day, but you avoid this by being careful. The same goes for weightlifting. Of course it's possible to hurt yourself or someone around you if you're not safe, but practising good technique and being self-aware will help to prevent any potential dangers.

Some people also think exercise on the whole causes joint issues, but the National Osteoporosis Foundation in the US and the NHS in the UK say

Leabharlanna Poibli Chathair Bhaile Átha Cliath
Dublin City Public Libraries

that when you exercise, you stimulate healthy fluid, which aids movement. Exercise also increases bone density and strength, meaning it fights diseases like osteoporosis.

MYTH: BEING HEAVY IS A BAD THING

As women, we have given way too much power to the weighing scales. I think it's time to throw them out. **The number on a scale does not reflect a true figure for the health of your body.** What is really amazing about gaining muscle is that your weight might go up slightly, but your shape will be smaller. The weighing scales also don't take account of water weight, bones, internal organs or lean muscle tissue, so stop focusing on the scales and start looking at yourself in the mirror.

MYTH: EXERCISING WILL MAKE YOUR BOOBS DISAPPEAR

Breast tissue is mostly made up of body fat. You should be proud and happy to see that being reduced and for your health to be improving. Getting fit and healthy will make you look better all over. In a dreamland we want to pick what to improve and what to lose, but that's not how it works. When you lose body fat, yes, your breast size will decrease, but I promise it won't be an issue when you see how amazing everything else looks.

MYTH: QUANTITY MATTERS MORE THAN QUALITY

Quality training is way more beneficial than the quantity of training you do. You could be in the gym for three hours messing around, taking

your time, chatting, looking at your phone or only training half-heartedly, or you could get into the gym and train your butt off for 45 minutes. Forty-five to 60 minutes is more than enough time to exercise. Training any longer will result in overtraining, meaning you are only counteracting your muscle gain. Get in, make it count and get out.

MYTH: THERE IS ONLY ONE WAY TO DO CARDIO

Cardiovascular activity comes in many forms: skipping, battle ropes, hill walking, sprints, you name it. You don't have to sit on a cross trainer for an hour to get enough cardio in. There is a huge range of fun ways to do cardio activity (see page 126 for more). **The main thing is to just get moving.**

MYTH: STRETCHING BEFORE EXERCISE IS IMPORTANT

This is an interesting one, actually. It has been proven in studies published in the *British Journal of Sports Medicine*, the *Strength and Conditioning Journal* and *Medicine and Science in Sports and Exercise* that stretching before exercise is not as beneficial for the body as warming up is. See page 84 for more information on warming up before exercise.

MYTH: LIFTING WEIGHTS ONLY BUILDS MUSCLE

Lifting weights offers huge benefits, including building muscle, but it also aids ongoing fat loss as a result of a boosted metabolism. After a weight-training session, the American Council on Exercise and the IDEA Health and Fitness Association say that your metabolism is active for over 24 hours after your workout, unlike cardio, which only burns calories during the time that you are exercising.

STRENGTH TRAINING AND CARDIO

There are four ways to do weight/strength training: body weight, machines, free weights and resistance. There is also a range of different ways to approach weightlifting, and this typically depends on your goals. So whether you are trying to slim down, tone up, build muscle, perk up or get strong, weight training does it all. It's a really effective way to exercise and the benefits are endless. Weight training is the stimulus for body change, so if you are looking to improve your shape, then start lifting.

Cardio, on the other hand, is the king of burning body fat and it also increases overall body performance, from speed to endurance. Cardiovascular activity is so much more than just slogging it out on a gym machine and it can be used in a much more clever way to help you reach your body and fitness goals. There are different techniques, from mixing up the intensity of your cardio to the duration.

Different approaches include:

- Low-intensity training (LIT), which means cardio activity done at a slow and steady pace, usually for 40–60 minutes.

- High-intensity training (HIT), where you aim to use explosive amounts of energy in short bursts, such as in 10-minute intervals.

- High-intensity interval training (HIIT), which means combining high-intensity cardio in explosive short bursts followed immediately by an active recovery period.

People tend to lean towards either weight training or cardiovascular activity, but **for maximum health and body benefits, you should combine them**.

WEIGHT TRAINING	CARDIO
• Weight training using machines	• Cardio training using machines
• Body weight exercises	• Jogging, running outside
• Weight training using free weights	• Plyometrics
• Resistance training	• High- or low-intensity cardio

THE TWO TYPES OF WEIGHTLIFTING MOVEMENTS

Weightlifting can be broken down into two specific categories: compound movements and isolated movements. Both serve different purposes within training, and both are important.

Compound movements are exercises that use more than one muscle in a movement. Typically one major muscle will do the work with the support of other, smaller muscles. For example, a squat is a compound movement because the majority of your lower body is used in performing this exercise, including your quads, glutes, hamstrings and lower back. Compounds burn more calories and fat than isolated exercise and also offer a better full-body workout.

Isolated movements are exercises that use only one muscle group in a movement or exercise. As the name suggests, you are isolating one muscle and it does all of the work. For example, a bicep curl, when performed using the right technique, only engages the bicep muscle and does not need the support of any other muscle to perform the movement. The benefits of isolated exercises are that they allow you to focus specifically on one area and make appropriate improvements.

For the best results, combine both compound and isolated exercises in your workouts, along with cardiovascular activity.

THE IMPORTANCE OF WARMING UP

Think about warming up like greasing a squeaky door, except that you're warming up your joints and getting the muscles ready to be used. People think that doing a couple of stretches before working out is enough, but warming up your muscles is much more beneficial. Although both would be ideal, **stretching involves preparing the joints for movement, whereas warming up activates the muscle and increases heart rate and body temperature**.

Before each workout, do 10 minutes of light cardio followed by five minutes of warm-up using light weights or even your own body weight. Doing this will help to prevent injury and also help to maximise results from your workout.

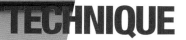

TECHNIQUE

I want you to understand the importance of training using proper technique rather than just going through a movement that isn't actually engaging the muscle. Training using correct technique means executing an exercise perfectly and avoiding injury. There is nothing more painful to watch than a novice taking on a deadlift with a bent-over back. The only thing that makes lifting weights dangerous is incorrect technique.

It's impossible to perform perfect technique from day one – it can take a while to understand and become the norm. Or if you've been training for weeks and weeks without seeing any results, it might be because you're not even engaging the muscles during exercise, and if you're not engaging them, then they are not being put under stress and therefore cannot change. When you're training, you should feel that exact muscle working; you shouldn't feel it in your joints and it shouldn't cause pressure. You need to think about the exercise and how it should work rather than simply just doing a movement for the sake of it. Engage your muscles and hit them properly. Lifting a weight with perfect technique is way more important than the amount of weight you lift.

Another big factor in training with good technique is supporting your spine, which usually means keeping your back position locked or concave, but never bent over.

TIPS ON TRAINING USING GOOD TECHNIQUE

- Always warm up before you start your workout.

- The only way to learn is by example, but that doesn't mean doing whatever your friend or other people are doing. Always consult a professional or somebody with a lot of experience. If you're a member of a gym, don't hesitate to ask the staff – that is what they are there for, and I promise they will be impressed that you asked.

- Start small. It isn't as easy to injure yourself using light weights and it's a great way to practise and familiarise yourself with the specific techniques of an exercise. Once you have mastered your form using the lighter weights, you can start considering increasing the weight.

- Be aware of your body. If something doesn't feel right, it probably isn't. You can help to avoid pain and potential injuries by being body conscious.

- I said it before, but I'll say it again – always support your spine. A spinal injury is no laughing matter. You can also use a weightlifting belt.

WHAT *NOT* TO DO WHEN YOU EXERCISE

There are many ways you can sabotage your fitness life. Let me point out a few of them so you can avoid them.

DON'T GO HELL FOR LEATHER FROM DAY ONE

It's not sustainable and certainly not realistic to train like a lunatic if you're new to all this. There is no point exercising twice a day, six days a week, straight away because you will just quickly burn yourself out and lose interest. Make this a fun and enjoyable transition into the fitness lifestyle. **Start off small and build yourself up as your knowledge of exercise builds.** According to my coach, Calin Brehaita, who has 23 years' experience as a personal trainer, and my own experience, here are some good guidelines for how often you should train.

BEGINNER	Three times a week for 45 minutes
INTERMEDIATE	Four to five times a week
ADVANCED	Five times a week or more

DON'T DO LAZY WORKOUTS

There is no such thing as a bad workout except the one you didn't do, but having said that, don't waste your time half-arsing a workout. Your time is valuable, so make the most of it. You are now an upcoming fitness star, so get motivated for your workout and work hard. **If you really want to see results, mediocre workouts won't cut it.** Don't cheat yourself.

DON'T QUIT BECAUSE IT'S HARD

There are going to be days that you are sore, tired or unmotivated. There will be early mornings when you'd rather stay in bed and dark, rainy evenings that you would prefer to sit on the couch watching TV. Or there will be times when you have to choose between a workout or going out. At these times, remember why you started. Even if you have a bad week and didn't exercise once, don't let it roll into the next week. Pick yourself back up. **Sometimes the hardest part is getting there, so just go.**

"'I'D RATHER BE SORE THAN SORRY."

TURN YOUR WEAKNESSES INTO A STRENGTH

We all have aspects of ourselves that we would love to change, but focusing on your weak points doesn't mean criticising yourself or putting yourself down. It means pinpointing the things you can improve on and overcoming your biggest challenges. For example, cardio has always been difficult for me due to my severe asthma, but I still maintain a regular cardio plan and I hope to do a marathon some day.

You can avoid your weak points, but then they will never get any better, so face them head on. Maybe there is a body part you hate training, or maybe your upper body needs more work than your lower body. Identify your weakness and then overcome it. Sometimes it's the most difficult and challenging aspects that change you the most and that will give you the biggest results. **The best things in life are the ones you have to work for, so turn your weakness into a strength.**

"WE GROW A LOT LIKE OUR MUSCLES DO — WHEN PUSHED TO THE LIMITS AND TORN OPEN, WE RECOVER AND GROW STRONGER THAN EVER BEFORE."

CONCLUSION

Exercise will help you, challenge you and make you healthier and happier. You should never feel ashamed or embarrassed to go to the gym or go out for a jog. You have every right to improve yourself, no matter what level you're at, and nobody has the right to make you feel otherwise. When it comes to exercise, remember that there is no one-size-fits-all format, so have fun experimenting in a safe way using proper technique and information.

Remember, too, that progress will take time, so don't give up. There is a future warrior in there that you will discover during each workout. One day you will look in the mirror or overcome an obstacle and you will be amazed at how far you have come. Don't compare your journey, your strength or your progress to anybody else. **Focus on you and focus on improving, not perfection.** Build your knowledge, ask questions, train with friends, get creative and enjoy it. Exercise is the fun part, so suck it up, work hard and smash those goals!

PART 02

THE
PLANS

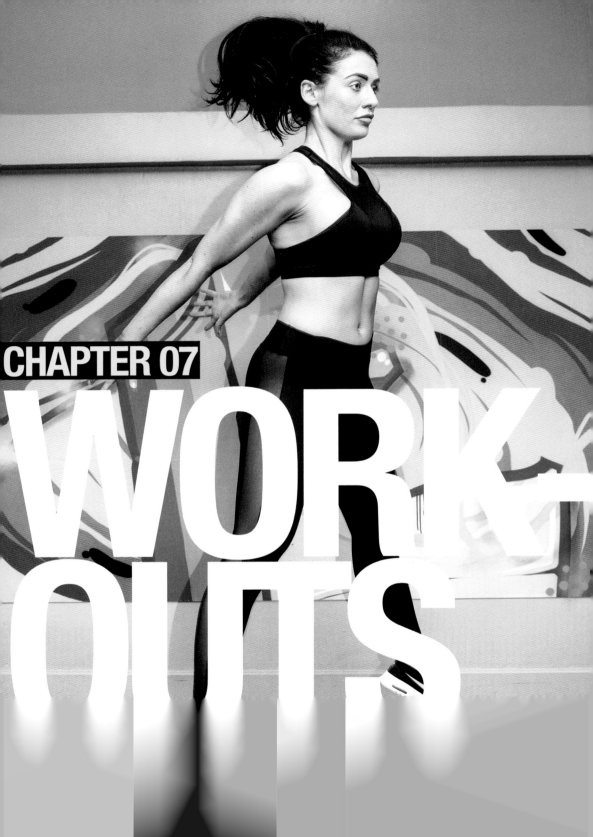

CHAPTER 07

WORK-OUTS

Exercise is one of my favourite things about fitness. I love nothing more than challenging myself in the gym, whether it's trying out new exercises, learning new tricks or just getting a sweat on. There are so many different styles of exercises and movements that target specific areas, so in this section I'm going to break down each body part for you to help you build your own knowledge. I'll also demonstrate some of my favourite exercise moves, but you can also check out my YouTube channel to see live demos of some of these exercises. I want to give you as much help as possible to achieve perfect technique when executing these exercises, because the correct technique is key.

MUSCLE GROUPS

GLUTES>

We all want a better posterior, and now more than ever it has become so trendy to have a big booty. But is it even possible? And if so, how do you do it?

It is absolutely possible to build your dream booty along with improving skin condition around the area, making things more perky, full and curvaceous. On the flip side, there is nothing worse for your booty than sitting on it too much.

On the whole, our glutes are underused and not trained either properly or enough. It's a large muscle group, so if you're serious about building size, then it will take a lot of work and it's important to train them correctly. We have all been brainwashed that squats are the booty saviour, when in fact they work your quads more than your glutes. Using a variety of exercises and combining compound and isolated movements will get better results. And don't forget to eat enough good food to fuel both intense booty workouts and recovery afterwards, which as you know is massively important for growth. Be sure to warm up and get your glutes activated prior to exercising.

Here are some badass exercises – literally! – for building the booty of your dreams.>>

"YOU DON'T GET THE BUM YOU WANT BY SITTING ON IT!"

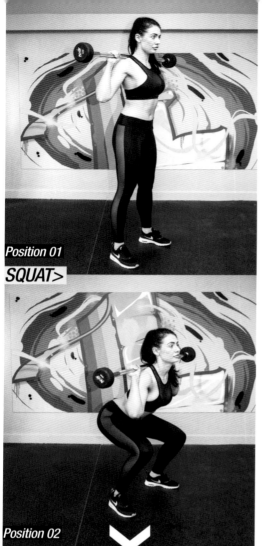

Position 01

SQUAT>

Position 02

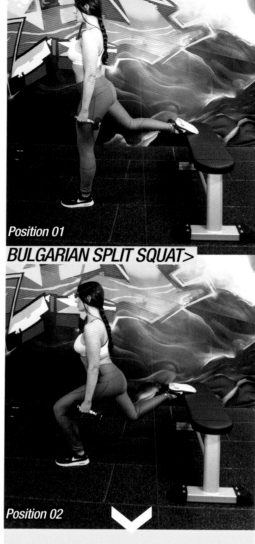

Position 01

BULGARIAN SPLIT SQUAT>

Position 02

> The squat is the ultimate exercise that EVERYONE should have in their programme. It's the king of compound movements. This exercise burns calories like no other and works both the glutes and the quadriceps. You can try it without any weight to start off with or something light like a barbell that you're comfortable lifting. You may want to use a spotter to help you out.

Standing with your feet roughly hip width apart, hold a barbell (if using) across your traps, gripping it with your palms facing away from your body (Position 01). Begin to lower yourself, bending your knees and keeping your back and spine as straight as possible (Position 02), before pushing back up to standing, and repeat. Let your legs do the work and focus on keeping your knees roughly in line with your feet.

> For this exercise, the only equipment you need is a free bench. Stand with your back to a bench roughly three feet away, feet shoulder width apart, and rest the front of your right foot on the bench behind you (Position 01). Take a couple of minutes to find your balance - try looking straight ahead and focusing on one point. Standing nice and tall, begin to bend your left leg, stretching out your glute slowly (Position 02). Be sure not to touch your right knee off the floor. Then push yourself back up, focusing on your glutes and quads. Repeat on your left leg.

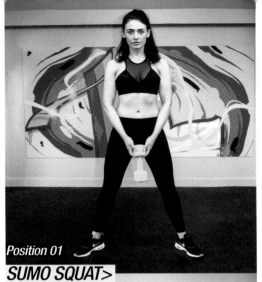

Position 01

SUMO SQUAT>

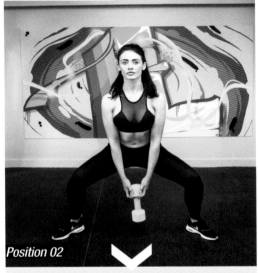

Position 02

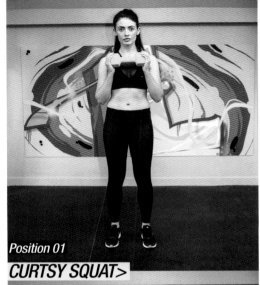

Position 01

CURTSY SQUAT>

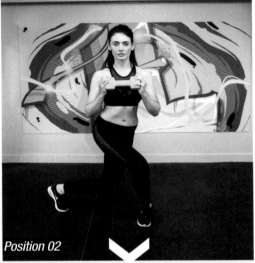

Position 02

> This is one of my favourite exercises at the minute – I use a long bar and more of a deadlift technique, but for now I will show you a super easy version using a dumbbell. The major difference with this and the classic squat (page 92) is that your stance is much wider and your toes point outwards. Using a dumbbell that you're comfortable lifting helps you to maintain your balance and stay central.

Start with a wide stance, holding one end of the dumbbell with both hands and letting it hang (Position 01). Begin to lower yourself until your quads are almost parallel with the floor and you feel a big stretch in the glutes (Position 02). Using your heels and glutes, drive yourself back up to standing and repeat.

> Start standing up tall, with your feet shoulder width apart, holding a dumbbell you're comfortable lifting between your hands (Position 01). Next, lower your right leg behind your body, taking a big step out to the left and bending both knees as if you're doing a curtsy (Position 02). Push back up, focusing on your quads and glutes. Repeat the move using your left leg. You can make this exercise more difficult by adding additional weight. This is such a fun exercise!

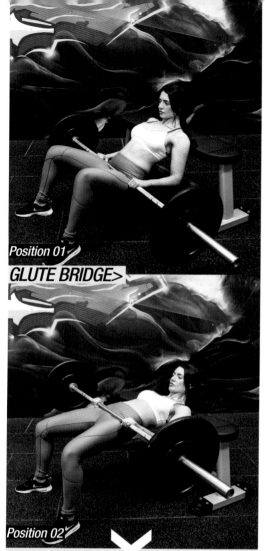

Position 01

GLUTE BRIDGE>

Position 02

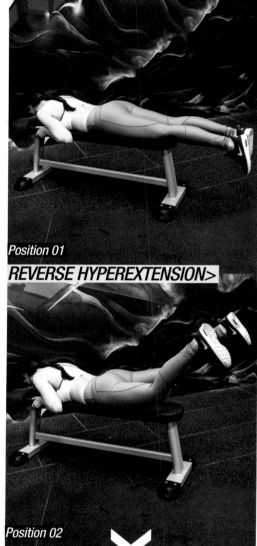

Position 01

REVERSE HYPEREXTENSION>

Position 02

> When it comes to building glutes, this exercise is king. There are many different variations on the basic movement, including using a leg extension machine, a smith machine and even a resistance loop (page 131). For this version, you will need a barbell (with a weight appropriate to you) and a bench. Try the movement without the barbell first and ask a friend to spot you.

With your back rested on the bench, rest the barbell directly over your hips with a nice firm grip. Keep your legs shoulder width apart (Position 01). Then raise the weight by thrusting your hips to the ceiling and squeezing your glute muscles. Pause at the top, squeezing your bum as much as possible (Position 02), then begin to lower your bum back to the floor nice and slowly, and repeat without resting.

> This is a super movement that I love to do either before a big glutes session to activate the muscle or after as a finisher. All you need to do is lie with your stomach flat on a bench, holding it firmly on either side with your legs flat behind you (Position 01). Begin to raise your heels to the ceiling, squeezing the glutes as much as possible (Position 02). As you raise your legs, start to spread them slightly, to make sure to target your gluteus maximus, and then repeat.

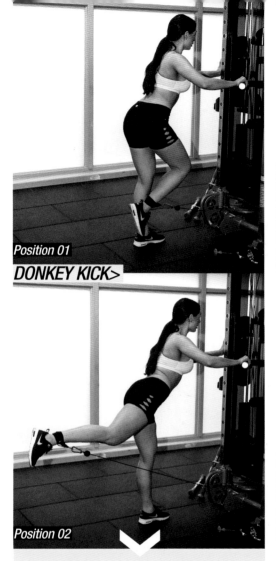

Position 01

DONKEY KICK>

Position 02

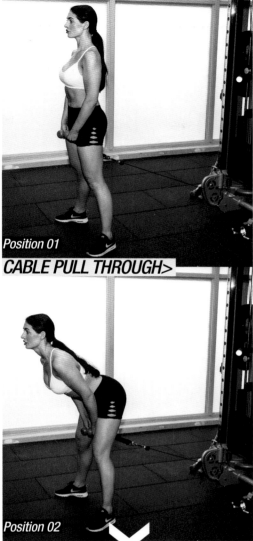

Position 01

CABLE PULL THROUGH>

Position 02

> The donkey kick is a great glute exercise that can be performed in many different ways. Here I am going to show you my personal favourite – using a cable machine.

Securing an ankle attachment around your right ankle, set the weight on the tower of the cable machine to the weight you're capable of lifting. Stand about two or three feet in front of the tower. Use your two hands to hold on to it in front of you (Position 01). Begin to kick back using the leg attached to the cable, driving with your heels and targeting your glute (Position 02). Then slowly bring the knee back towards the tower and repeat. You will see my knees are slightly bent through the entire motion. Be sure to keep your core engaged.

> For this exercise, you will need one side of a cable machine and a rope attachment, setting the height to the lowest point and choosing a weight you're capable of lifting. Stand two to three feet away from the cable machine, with your back to the tower. Hold both sides of the rope with your palms facing each other. You should be standing directly over the pulley, holding it between your legs (Position 01). Begin to lower your torso, allowing the pulley to literally pull you back until your torso is almost parallel to the floor (Position 02). Don't worry if you can't come down too low – this will all depend on the flexibility of your hamstrings. The most important thing is that you feel a big stretch in the hamstrings and lower glutes. Then thrust your hips and the pulley back into standing, squeezing your glutes, and repeat.

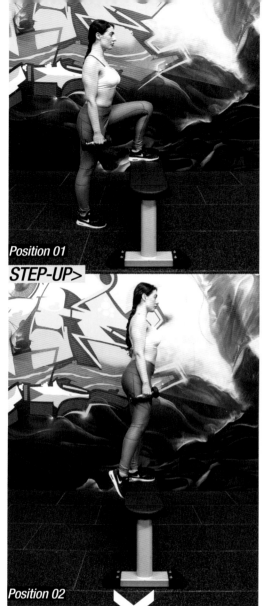

Position 01

STEP-UP>

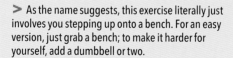

Position 02

> As the name suggests, this exercise literally just involves you stepping up onto a bench. For an easy version, just grab a bench; to make it harder for yourself, add a dumbbell or two.

Place the bench in front of you and step up with your left foot, using your heel to lift you and your glute (Position 01). Pressing into your left foot, lift yourself up onto the bench, leaving your right foot hanging down (Position 02). Slowly lower yourself back down and repeat.

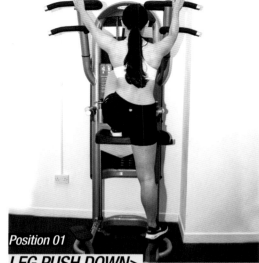

Position 01

LEG PUSH DOWN>

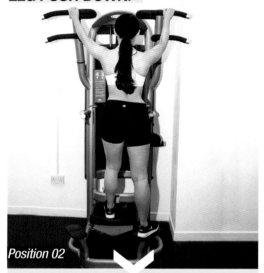

Position 02

> For this exercise, you will need to find the assisted pull up machine in your gym. Stand on the machine, facing it, and set the weight appropriate to you. Use the bars above you to hold yourself with a grip wider than shoulder width apart. Place your right foot on the pad (Position 01). Begin to push down, using your glute and focusing on driving the heel down (Position 02). Repeat as required, then switch sides.

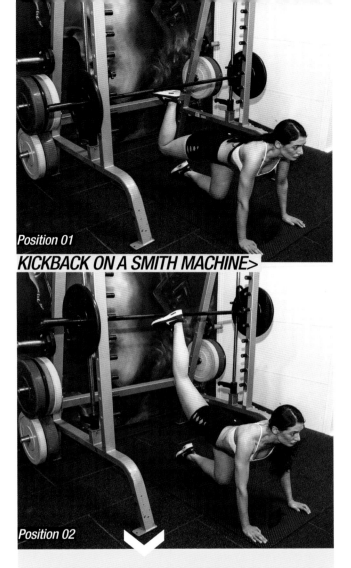

Position 01

KICKBACK ON A SMITH MACHINE>

Position 02

> Kneeling on a mat with your hands flat on the ground or leaning on your forearms, put your right foot behind you, touching the smith machine. Make sure the weight is set to your preference. Your right quad should be parallel to the floor (Position 01). Begin to push the smith machine bar directly up, using your leg and quads to drive the bar upward (Position 02). You may find it handy to have a spotter to help you unclip the bar or you may prefer to use a lighter weight. When you extend your leg as far as possible, begin to lower it back down, not letting your knee touch the ground, and repeat.

HAMSTRINGS>

Did you know that your hamstrings play a hugely important role in improving your booty? All four elements of your legs are connected – glutes, hamstrings, quads and calves – so it's essential to make time for each and every one of them. If one area is weaker, it will affect your progress with the rest. Having strong hamstrings also maintains strong knees and balance.

Here are some of my favourite hamstring exercises.>>

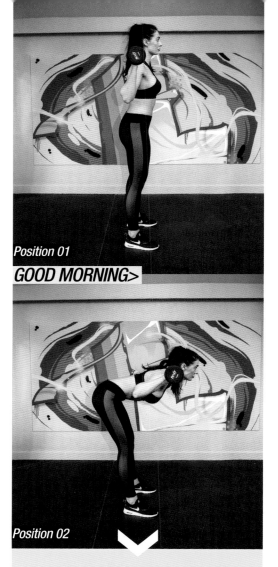

Position 01

GOOD MORNING>

Position 02

> Standing nice and tall, with your feet hip width apart, position the barbell (with whatever weight suits you) to rest on your traps, gripping the barbell tightly with your palms facing away from your body (Position 01). Begin to lean your torso forward by bending from the hips, coming down until the front of your body is almost parallel to the floor and focusing on stretching your hamstrings (Position 02). Then bring your body back upright, constantly squeezing your glutes, and repeat.

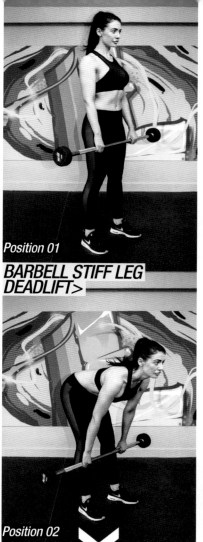

Position 01

BARBELL STIFF LEG DEADLIFT>

Position 02

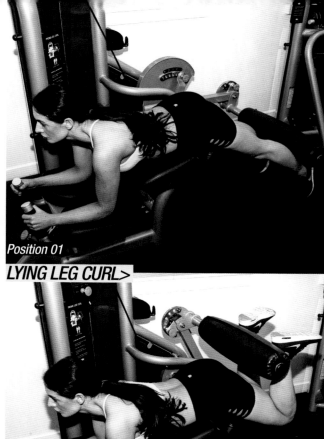

Position 01

LYING LEG CURL>

Position 02

> To start, stand tall and let the barbell (with a weight you can lift) hang in front of you, holding it shoulder width apart with your palms facing your body (Position 01). Begin to lower your pelvis slowly, sticking your bum out and keeping your back nice and strong. Your torso should be roughly parallel to the floor as the barbell lowers towards your toes (Position 02). If your flexibility only allows you to come to your knees, that's no problem – just focus on stretching the hamstrings and be very careful not to arch your back.

> Machines are super for doing weights because you can't really go wrong. For this exercise, all you need to do is jump onto the leg curl machine, with your stomach lying flat on the bench (Position 01). Make sure you've set your weight appropriately and adjusted the leg pad to a suitable level on your legs. With your legs fully extended, begin to curl your legs, lifting the pad towards your bum and keeping your toes straight (Position 02). I like to point my toes slightly outwards during the curling movement in this exercise as I find it's easier on my knees, so try both and find out what suits you. Once the pad tips your bum, slowly lower it back down and then repeat.

QUADS>

As the name suggests, the quads are comprised of four different muscles. Training your quads is usually the most daunting day of them all – yes, I'm talking about the dreaded leg day. But if you're serious about your training, then you are going to have to get in there and lift like the men. Training quads not only gives you sexy, toned legs, but it also boosts your metabolism and burns up calories like an oven.

Here are some great leg exercises that you should try out.>>

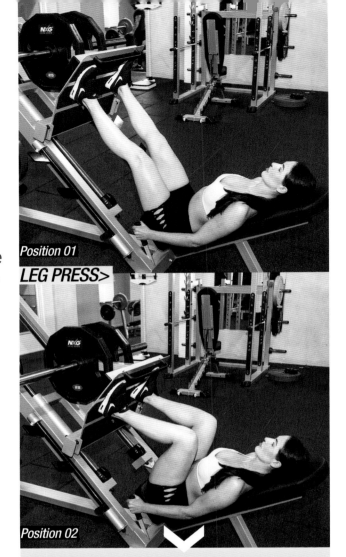

Position 01

LEG PRESS>

Position 02

> Use a leg press machine for this exercise. Lie on your back, with your legs hip width apart and resting on the machine. Make sure you've set the weight to one that suits you and adjusted the back pad so that you're comfortable. Start by slowly lowering the weight towards your body (Position 01). Then extend your legs upwards, driving through your feet (Position 02), and repeat. Use a safety clip during this exercise to prevent any accidents.

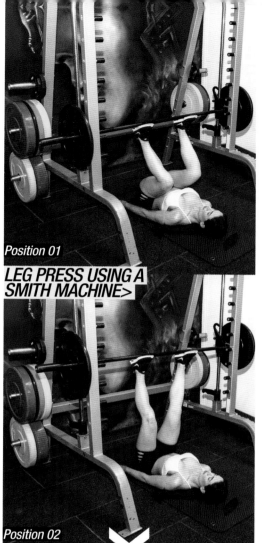

Position 01

LEG PRESS USING A SMITH MACHINE>

Position 02

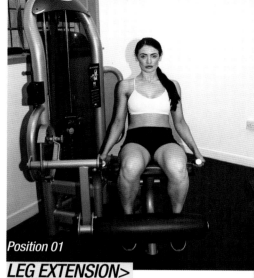

Position 01

LEG EXTENSION>

Position 02

> The smith machine leg press is exactly the same as the leg press machine version, except you don't lie on the machine in this version. Instead, start by lying flat on your back (using a mat for comfort). Set the weight on the smith machine bar to one that suits you and set it two or three feet away from your body. Place both of your feet on the bar, roughly hip width apart, with your knees slightly bent. Then lower the bar towards your body so that your knees almost touch your chest (Position 01). Then drive the bar upwards until your legs are fully extended (Position 02). As with the leg press machine, always use a safety clip during this exercise to prevent any accidents.

> For this exercise, you need to use the leg extension machine. Set the seat to suit you, with the pads on your lower legs, just above the ankles (Position 01). Make sure the weight is suitable for you. With your toes pointing forward and holding the handles beside you, drive the pads upwards until your legs are fully extended (Position 02). Focus on your quads and enjoy the burn.

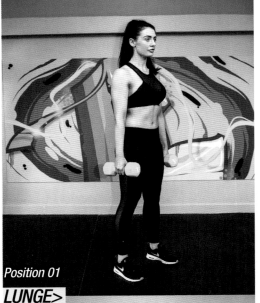

Position 01

LUNGE>

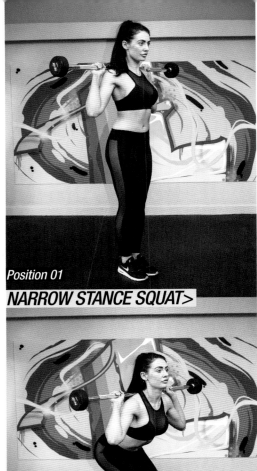

Position 01

NARROW STANCE SQUAT>

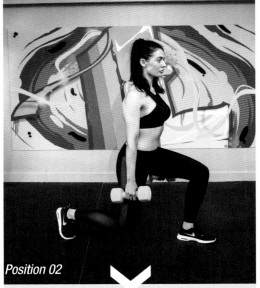

Position 02

Position 02

> Stand up tall, with your feet hip width apart (Position 01). If you're feeling strong, add a barbell or dumbbells in each hand, but feel free to try this exercise using just your body weight – you'll still feel it! Step forward with your left leg and lower your body with your hips, bringing your right knee towards the floor (Position 02). Find your balance and take it slow. Make sure not to let your right knee come past your right toes. Push back up to standing and repeat on the other side.

> This is exactly like the classic squat (page 92) except you keep both legs together through the entire exercise. Start standing upright, with your feet together (Position 01). Then lower yourself using your hips and bum, keeping your torso upright (Position 02). Push yourself back to standing and repeat. It's as simple as that! For added difficulty, try doing it with a barbell (with a weight that suits you), as I am in the photo, or using a smith machine.

CALVES>

When you wear a dress, the first thing people will spot is a great pair of pins. Training your calves is easy and it takes very little to stimulate them to change, so there's a lot of potential for improvement. A lot of women tend to avoid this area because they don't see any issues with their calves, but a true fitness queen will target and engage every muscle group.

Stronger calves mean stronger legs.>>

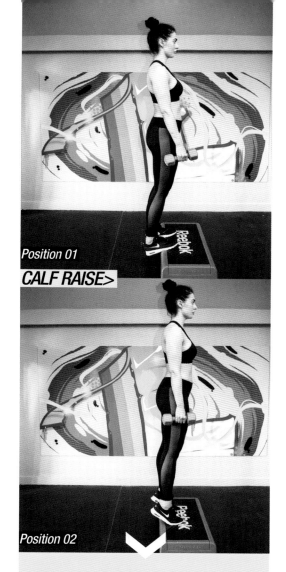

Position 01

CALF RAISE>

Position 02

> This calf raise can be done in so many ways that it's the only calf exercise I've included in *BYOB*. Once you get the basic technique sorted, you can experiment with other positions.

Start by standing on a small step with your toes pointing forward and your heels hanging slightly back off the step (Position 01). Slowly begin to raise your body, using your calf muscles to drive the body up (Position 02). Lower back to the starting position and then repeat – it's that simple!

When you're comfortable with the technique, try a couple on one leg (single leg calf raises) and some with your toes pointed in or outwards. If you're feeling adventurous, try and find the calf raise machine in your gym.

ABS>

The abs are a tricky area for most women. Many women train and train and train without seeing results, but as we discussed earlier, your ab development could potentially be hidden underneath a layer of body fat. That being said, you should always continue to train them because as your body fat drops around the area, some great developments will come through. Having a strong core is essential for stability and for protecting your organs, and it also helps you to maintain good posture.

Here are some brilliant ab exercises.>>

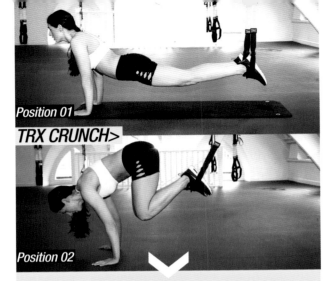

Position 01

TRX CRUNCH>

Position 02

> Begin in a suspended plank position, with your hands directly in front of you and both feet in the TRX loops (Position 01). Next, bring your knees forward until they are at a 90-degree angle to your body (Position 02). Hold briefly, then return to Position 01 and repeat.

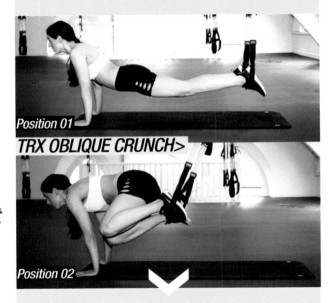

Position 01

TRX OBLIQUE CRUNCH>

Position 02

> Begin in a suspended plank position, with your hands directly in front of you and both feet in the TRX loops (Position 01). Next, twist your body as you bring your knees towards your elbows (Position 02). Hold briefly, then return to Position 01 and repeat.

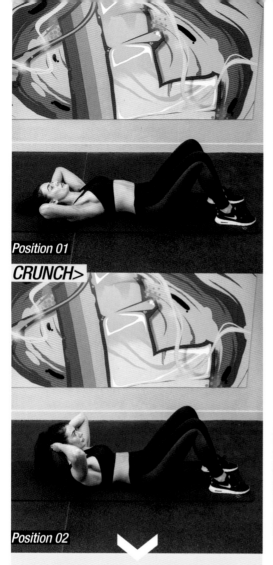

Position 01

CRUNCH>

Position 02

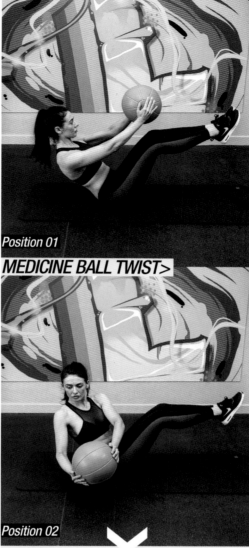

Position 01

MEDICINE BALL TWIST>

Position 02

> Using a mat behind your back for crunches will help keep you comfortable. Lie with your back flat on the mat, with your feet roughly hip width apart, your knees bent and the soles of your feet firmly flat on the floor. You can position your arms whatever way you like – crossed over your chest or behind your head (Position 01). Begin to crunch the body forward, lifting your shoulders and keeping your arms aligned with your head (Position 02). Then slowly lower to the start position and repeat. It's a pretty small movement but a very effective one.

> Also called the Russian twist, you can use a medicine ball, dumbbell or plate for this exercise. Keeping your bum on the mat, lift your torso to 45 degrees and your legs to 45 degrees, making your body into a V shape. Holding the weight, extend your arms directly out in front of you (Position 01). Twist your torso around to your right, so that the weight is almost touching the ground (Position 02). Then return to centre and repeat on the left side.

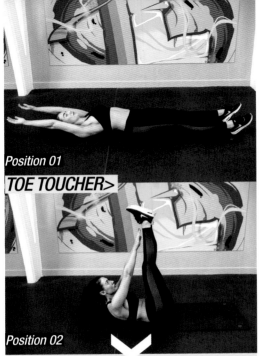

Position 01

TOE TOUCHER>

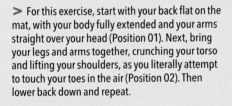

Position 02

> For this exercise, start with your back flat on the mat, with your body fully extended and your arms straight over your head (Position 01). Next, bring your legs and arms together, crunching your torso and lifting your shoulders, as you literally attempt to touch your toes in the air (Position 02). Then lower back down and repeat.

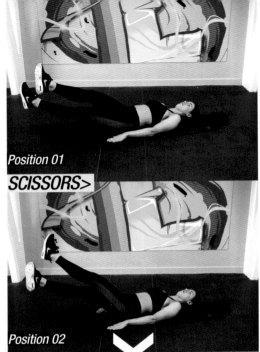

Position 01

SCISSORS>

Position 02

> Lying on the floor with your back flat on the mat, place both hands palms down directly beside your body. Lift your legs roughly 45 degrees from the floor and cross your right leg over your left (Position 01). For this exercise, you simply alternate crossing one leg over the other in a scissor motion, bringing your left leg over the right, then the right over the left (Position 02).

PLANK>

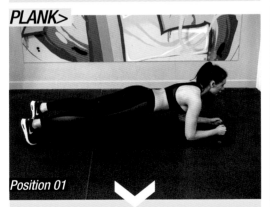

Position 01

> Using your toes and forearms, balance yourself with your body facing the ground and your head looking forward (Position 01). Keep your body straight and hold yourself in this position for as long as possible.

SIDE PLANK>

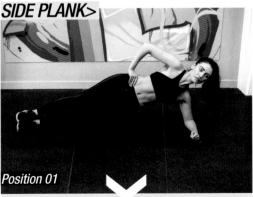

Position 01

> This is the exact same as the original plank, except you turn to the side and support your body using one arm at a time and the sides of your feet (Position 01).

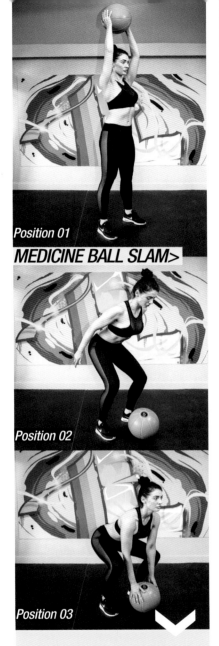

Position 01

MEDICINE BALL SLAM>

Position 02

Position 03

> This explosive exercise doesn't just torch calories – it works both your abs and back. Stand up tall, holding a medicine ball directly above your head with your feet shoulder width apart (Position 01). Slam the ball with full intensity onto the ground (Position 02). Then squat down to pick up the ball (Position 03) and repeat.

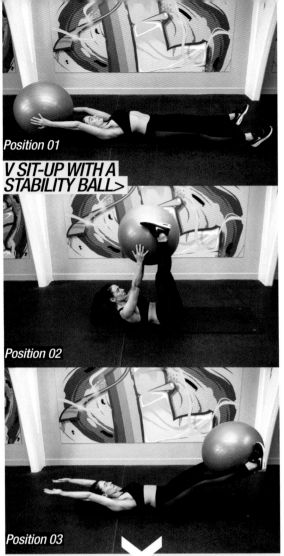

Position 01

V SIT-UP WITH A STABILITY BALL>

Position 02

Position 03

> For this exercise, also called a hand to feet ball pass, you'll need a mat and a stability ball. Lying with your back on the ground with your body fully extended, hold the ball in your hands above your head (Position 01). Next, begin to lift your legs towards your body and at the same time bring your arms and the ball to meet them (Position 02). Grasp the stability ball between your feet and lower it back to the floor, stretching out your lower abs and bringing your arms back up above your head (Position 03). Then do it in the opposite direction, passing the ball back from your feet to your hands. It's easier than it looks (I promise!) and so much fun.

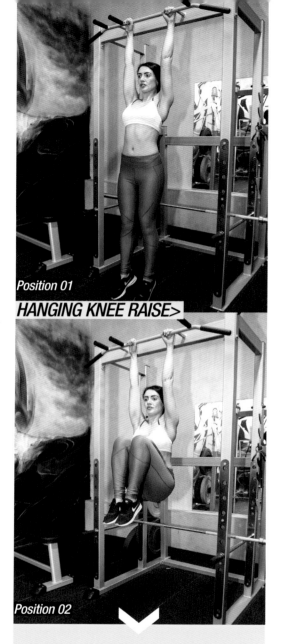

Position 01

HANGING KNEE RAISE>

Position 02

> Start by hanging from a chin-up bar by your arms, which should be slightly wider than shoulder width part, with your legs hanging (Position 01). Next, raise your knees towards your body, as high as they can go (Position 02). Then lower back down and repeat. If you find these easy, why not try the more advanced version, hanging leg raises, where you lift your legs straight out in front of you?

BICEPS AND TRICEPS>

Do you want to fight bingo wings and keep your arms toned and tight? Smashing bis and tris (biceps and triceps) isn't just for men. It's time to embrace the power in your arms and get your very own lady guns. Your arms need to be strong to lift, so don't be afraid to invest in them. And don't worry, women can't get giant arms – we simply don't produce the testosterone necessary to do it. What you will get, however, is sexy, shapely arms that will look amazing when you wear a vest or a dress.

Here are some great arm-toning exercises.>>

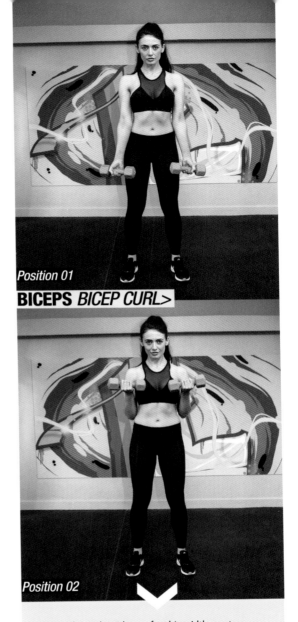

Position 01

BICEPS *BICEP CURL>*

Position 02

> Stand upright with your feet hip width apart, your core engaged and a dumbbell that is a suitable weight for you in each hand. The dumbbells should be by your side, with your palms facing forward (Position 01). Raise both dumbbells towards your body until they are almost at your shoulders, contracting your bicep (Position 02). Then lower them back down to the original position and repeat. Use control at all times and focus on the muscle you are working, your bicep. Perform the move nice and slow, squeezing the bicep constantly. For a resistance variation on the bicep curl, check out page 129.

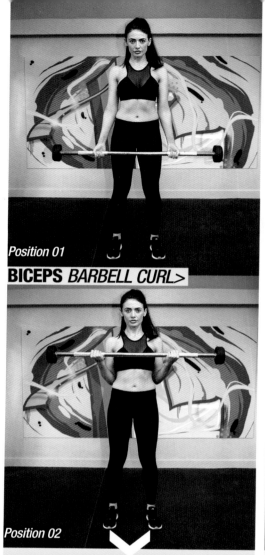

Position 01

BICEPS *BARBELL CURL>*

Position 02

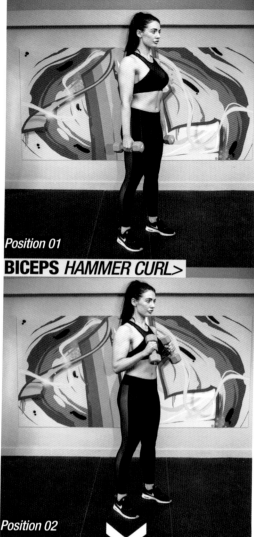

Position 01

BICEPS *HAMMER CURL>*

Position 02

> Stand upright with your feet hip width apart and your core engaged, in the same stance as the bicep curl (page 109). Hold the barbell (with a weight that suits you) with your arms extended downwards and your palms facing forward (Position 01). This exercise should be performed with your elbows controlling the entire range of motion, so keep them locked by your side. Next, lift the barbell slowly towards your body (Position 02). As you raise the barbell, keep your biceps contracted; the same goes when you lower the barbell back down. Keep your bicep under tension and control the movement. You can also do this exercise lying on a bench or using a cable bar.

> Stand upright with a dumbbell you're comfortable lifting in either hand, held beside your body with your palms facing inwards towards the side of your legs (Position 01). As in the other bicep exercises, keep your elbows locked when performing a hammer curl. Raise the dumbbells towards your chest, contracting your bicep while lifting the weight upwards (Position 02). Then lower and repeat.

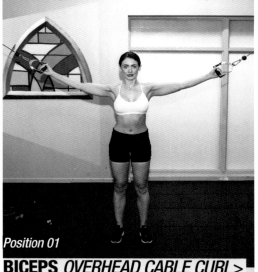

Position 01

BICEPS *OVERHEAD CABLE CURL>*

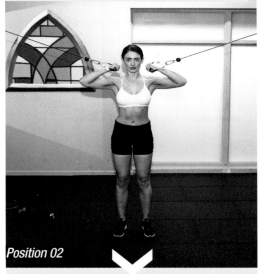

Position 02

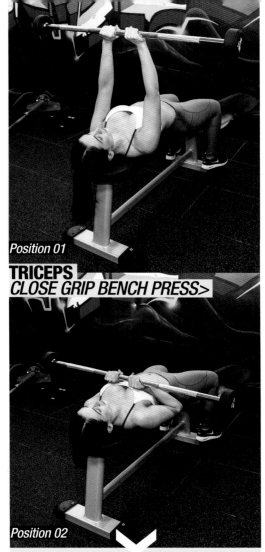

Position 01

TRICEPS
CLOSE GRIP BENCH PRESS>

Position 02

> For this exercise, you will need access to the cable machine at your gym. Set the height at both sides of the machine to a level that is slightly higher than shoulder level, and make sure the weight on both sides is set to a manageable level. Standing in the centre of the machine, hold a handle in each hand, with your palms facing the ceiling and your arms fully extended (Position 01). Bring the handles towards you until your forearms and biceps meet (Position 02). Then release outwards and repeat.

> Start by lying with your back flat on a bench and your hands locked around the barbell (with a suitable weight) above you. Extend your arms straight above you, shoulder width apart (Position 01). Begin to lower the barbell towards your body until it touches your chest (Position 02). Be sure to keep your elbows beside your body so that you target your triceps. Then extend upwards again, constantly focusing on using your triceps, and repeat. This exercise is a great one to try with a spotter, like a friend or a gym buddy.

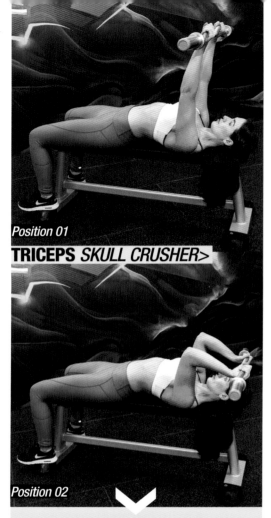

Position 01

TRICEPS *SKULL CRUSHER>*

Position 02

> Lying with your back flat on a bench, hold your barbell (with a suitable weight) above you using a closed grip, as in the close grip bench press (page 111). This means your hands should hold the barbell shoulder width apart (Position 01). Begin to lower the barbell slowly towards your forehead, bending at your elbows to lower the barbell 90 degrees and keeping your shoulders and elbows parallel (Position 02). Then straighten your arms and repeat. Take this exercise slow, starting off with a light weight, and be sure to stop before your touch your forehead.

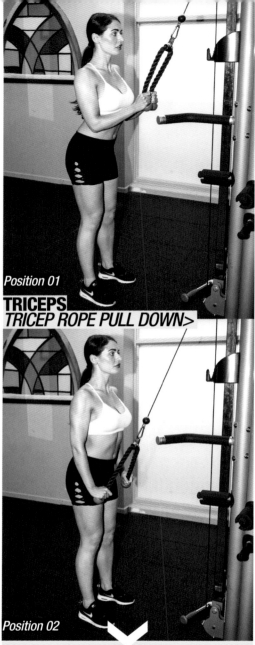

Position 01

TRICEPS
TRICEP ROPE PULL DOWN>

Position 02

> Using one side of the cable machine, clip a rope attachment to the hook. Standing up straight, hold the two sides of the rope with your palms facing each other and your arms bent (Position 01). Bring the rope down towards the front of your legs, using your forearms and constantly squeezing your triceps (Position 02). Then release the rope back up and repeat.

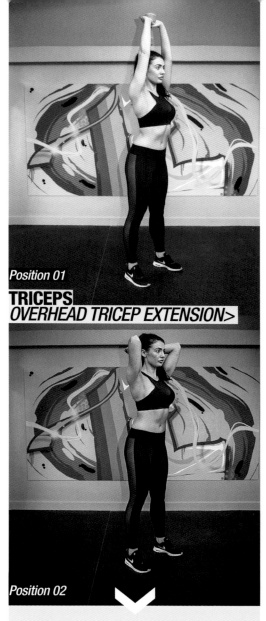

Position 01

TRICEPS
OVERHEAD TRICEP EXTENSION>

Position 02

> Standing upright with your feet shoulder width apart, grip one end of a dumbbell you're able to lift comfortably with both hands, with both thumbs around the dumbbell. Your palms should face the ceiling. Hold the dumbbell straight above your head (Position 01). Keep your arms beside your head and begin to lower the dumbbell, using your elbows. Lower the weight until your biceps touch your forearms, concentrating on your triceps (Position 02). Then extend your arms upwards and repeat.

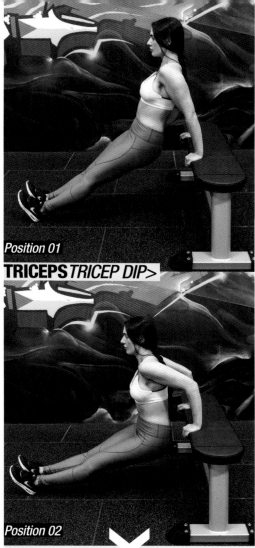

Position 01

TRICEPS *TRICEP DIP>*

Position 02

> This compound exercise is a real killer but it's an essential for banishing bingo wings and toning triceps and all you need is a bench. With your back to the bench, facing forward, grip the side of the bench (Position 01). Slowly lower yourself down, using your triceps (Position 02). Then push back up and repeat. You can also do this exercise using a tricep dip bar or a tricep machine, which can be found in most gyms. If you want to make it harder, rest a weight on your quads.

SHOULDERS>

Time to grow those boulder shoulders, ladies! Nothing is cooler than a strong set of delts. The benefits of training your upper body parts, like your shoulders and back, include better overall proportions and the appearance of a smaller waist. My shoulders are one of my favourite body parts to train. There is nothing I love more than showing off my shoulder gains in a selfie.

Here's how you can get boulder shoulders.>>

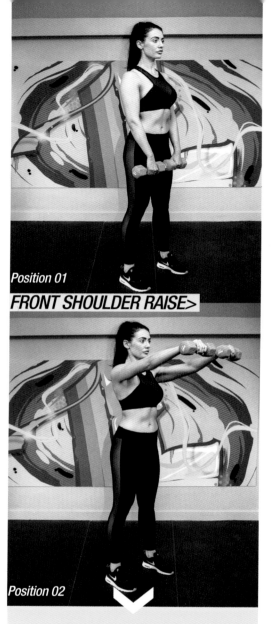

Position 01

FRONT SHOULDER RAISE>

Position 02

> Start by standing upright with a dumbbell of suitable weight for you in each hand, gripping them with your palms facing your quads (Position 01). Then it couldn't be more simple – raise the dumbbells straight ahead of you until they are in line with your shoulders (Position 02). Then lower and repeat. Remember, avoid swinging the dumbbells up – instead, use a slow controlled movement so that your shoulders do all the work.

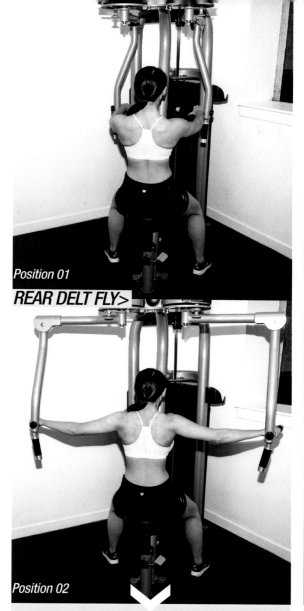

Position 01

REAR DELT FLY>

Position 02

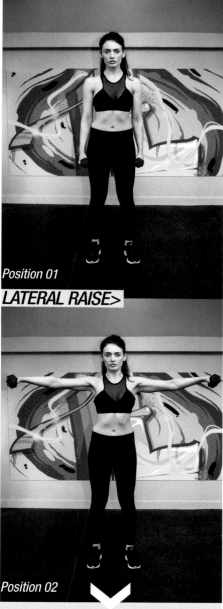

Position 01

LATERAL RAISE>

Position 02

> It's so important to target all areas of your delts and this exercise, sometimes called a reverse fly, is great for hitting the back of the shoulders. It can be done with a machine or with dumbbells, standing or using a bench. To use a machine, start by adjusting the bench position to suit you and setting the weight to a manageable level. Place your hands on the handles to begin (Position 01). Then bring the bars straight out to the side (Position 02). Return them to the centre, squeezing your delts slowly, and repeat. Make sure to focus on the back of your shoulders when doing this exercise and don't worry about having a slight bend in your elbows if you need it.

> The lateral raise is very similar to the front shoulder raise (page 114) except you raise the dumbbell out to the side instead of the front. Start by standing up straight with a dumbbell of an appropriate weight for you in each hand. Your palms should face towards your quads (Position 01). Then raise the dumbbell laterally, using a slow, controlled movement, until it reaches shoulder height (Position 02). Lower and repeat.

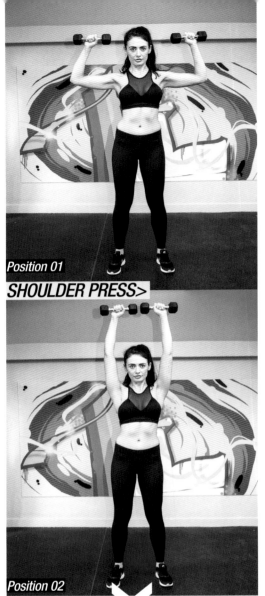

SHOULDER PRESS>

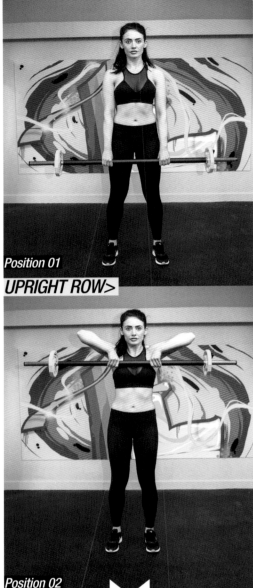

UPRIGHT ROW>

> Stand tall with feet shoulder width apart and a dumbbell of comfortable weight in each hand, palms facing away from your body and your core engaged. Start with your arms bent and the dumbbells in line with your head (Position 01). Then drive the dumbbells towards the ceiling, using your shoulders (Position 02). Bend your arms again and repeat. You can also perform this exercise sitting on a bench, with a Smith machine or using resistance cables (see page 130).

> Start by standing up tall, gripping a barbell you're comfortable lifting with your palms facing the front of your quads. Your grip should be roughly shoulder width apart with your back straight and your core engaged (Position 01). Begin to lift the barbell upwards, driving your elbows up to the same level as your head and using your shoulders to power the motion (Position 02). Then lower back down and repeat. The best way to nail this exercise is to aim to bring your elbows high. You could also try this exercise with a resistance band with handles, a smith machine, dumbbells or even a cable machine.

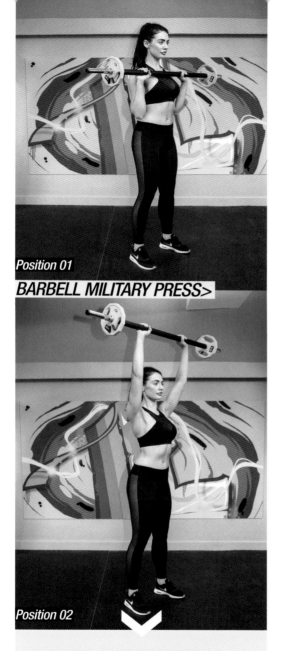

Position 01

BARBELL MILITARY PRESS>

Position 02

> Standing upright, hold a barbell that you are comfortable lifting with your palms facing away from your body. Both hands should be a little wider than shoulder width apart. To start, hold the barbell just above your chest (Position 01). Next, drive the barbell over your head and slightly forward, so that the barbell doesn't end up directly above your head but instead just ahead of it (Position 02). Then lower and repeat.

CHEST>

A lot of women never train their chest, to their detriment. Every body part is connected and it's crucial to strengthen all aspects of your body, not just one or two parts.

If you want to improve strength in your upper body and avoid having body imbalances, then tone that chest.>>

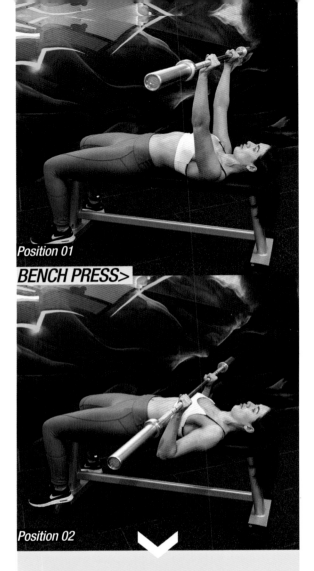

Position 01

BENCH PRESS>

Position 02

> This is a great compound exercise that women typically avoid, but shouldn't. It not only target the chest, but works your shoulders and triceps as well. Start by lying flat on a bench, holding a barbell of a suitable weight for you directly over the middle of your chest. Your grip should be wider than shoulder width apart (Position 01). Begin to lower the barbell down towards you until you tip your chest (Position 02). Then drive the bar back upwards and repeat. Why not try this exercise with a friend or spotter?

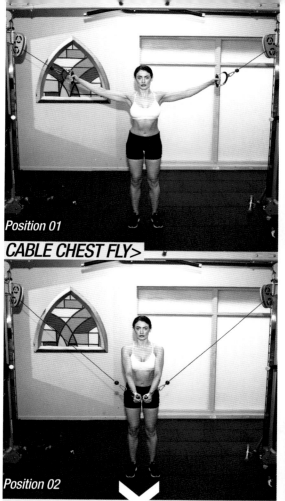

Position 01

CABLE CHEST FLY>

Position 02

> Using a cable machine, attach a handle to each side. Set the weight to something you feel comfortable with – always try something light until you feel comfortable with the movement. Position the level to roughly the highest point and stand directly between the two towers. Grip both handles with your palms facing away from the body. Take a small step forward and lean your torso slightly forward (Position 01). Begin to bring both handles together until they meet, being sure to keep a slight bend in your elbow (Position 02). Then return your arms to the starting position and repeat. You should feel a nice stretch in your chest during this exercise.

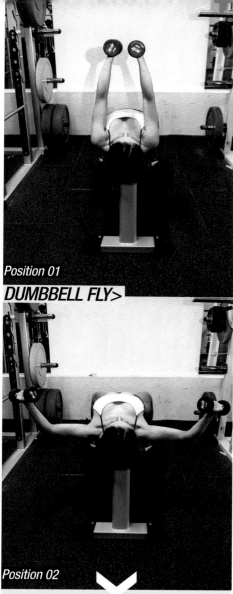

Position 01

DUMBBELL FLY>

Position 02

> Lying with your back flat on a bench, hold a dumbbell of suitable weight in each hand directly over your chest. Grip them with your palms facing each other (Position 01). Begin to lower both dumbbells, bending your elbows until you feel that stretch in your bicep (Position 02). Then lift your arms back to centre and repeat.

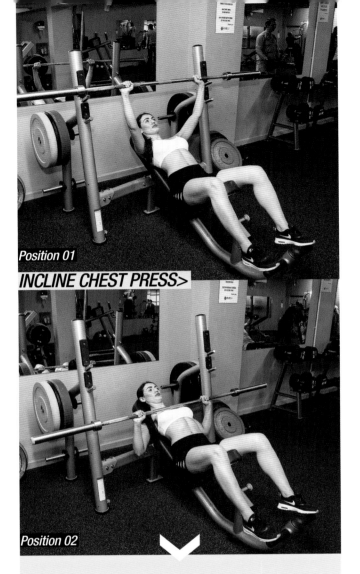

Position 01

INCLINE CHEST PRESS>

Position 02

> The incline chest press is very similar to the standard bench press (page 118) except the bench is positioned on an incline. It's a super move for hitting your upper chest area. With your back flat on the incline bench and your feet firmly placed on the floor, hold a barbell with a suitable weight directly above you, with your grip wider than shoulder width apart. If you're using a weight rack, lift the barbell off and straighten your arms (Position 01). Then lower the barbell towards you, slightly arching your back, and bring the barbell down to your upper chest (Position 02). Then bring the bar back up above you and repeat. You could also try this with dumbbells, on a cable machine or on a smith machine.

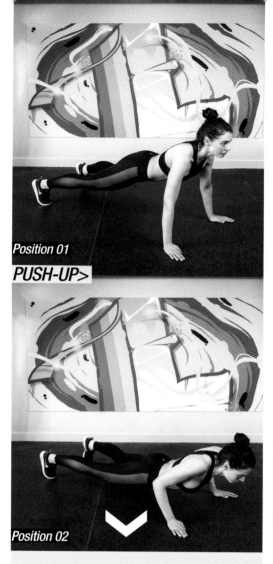

Position 01

PUSH-UP>

Position 02

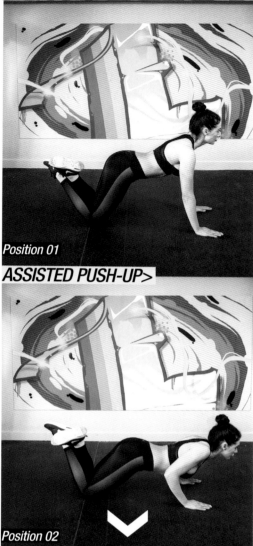

Position 01

ASSISTED PUSH-UP>

Position 02

> The push-up is a must – it's definitely not an exercise to be feared. Start by balancing on your palms and your toes, with your body extended in a straight line. Your hands should be a little wider than shoulder width apart (Position 01). Next, lower yourself slowly to the ground until your chest almost touches the floor (Position 02). Then push yourself back upright and repeat. If you find this a little challenging, try the assisted push-up instead.

> The assisted push-up is the same as the standard push-up except you balance on your knees instead of your toes. Start by balancing on your palms and your knees, with your legs crossed at the ankle. Your back should be straight and your weight should be over your hands (Position 01). Next, lower yourself to the ground, bending your elbows (Position 02). Then push yourself back up and repeat.

BACK>

There is nothing better than a session with pull-ups and deadlifts. It's a seriously tough day in the gym that burns bags of calories, and it's one of my favourite workout days. This is also the key area for producing that tiny waist and V shape that everyone wants.

Here are some wicked back exercises that you should try.>>

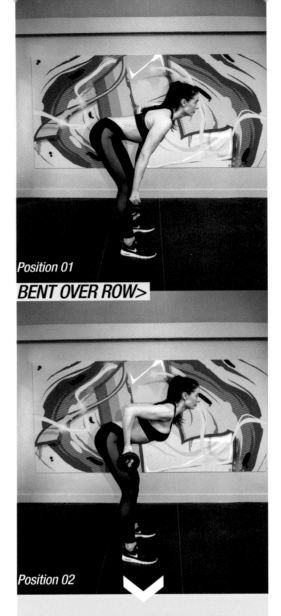

Position 01

BENT OVER ROW>

Position 02

> Keeping your back straight, bend your body forward, with your feet firmly on the ground about shoulder width apart. Hold a barbell with an appropriate weight with your arms extended towards the ground. Your palms can either face towards or away from your body (Position 01). Facing forward, begin to lift the barbell towards your body until your elbows are above your back (Position 02). Then lower down and repeat. Be sure to keep your arms close to your body and focus on the muscles you are working: your back.

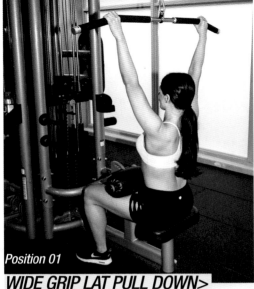

Position 01

WIDE GRIP LAT PULL DOWN>

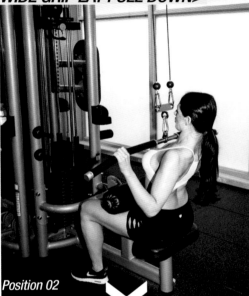

Position 02

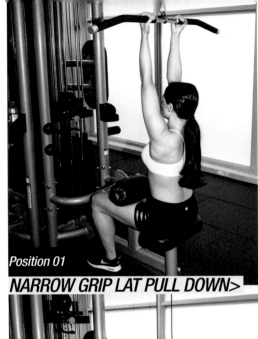

Position 01

NARROW GRIP LAT PULL DOWN>

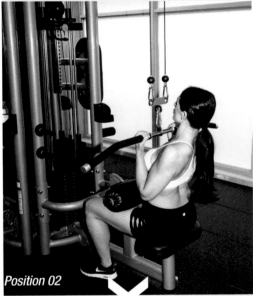

Position 02

> Using a lat pull down machine, set the knee pads to an appropriate level and choose a weight that's suitable for you. Sit into the machine, facing the bar. Hold the bar above your head, gripping it slightly wider than shoulder width apart with your palms facing away from your body (Position 01). Begin to lower the bar, leaning back slightly to allow room for the bar to touch your upper chest area (Position 02). Don't forget to squeeze those back muscles. Then release and repeat. You could also do this exercise using a bench or a cable machine.

> The narrow grip lat pull down is similar to the wide grip one – just the hand position is different. In this exercise, your palms face your body as you grip underneath the bar. Make sure the machine is set up correctly, with the appropriate weight and comfortable pads. Sit into position, holding onto the bar above your head with your hands in an under grip closer than shoulder width apart (Position 01). Then do the exact same as in the wide grip lat pull down – bring your elbows past your body, keeping your arms tucked in and squeezing your back muscles (Position 02). Then release and repeat.

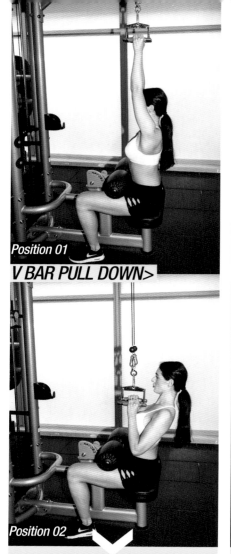

Position 01

V BAR PULL DOWN>

Position 02

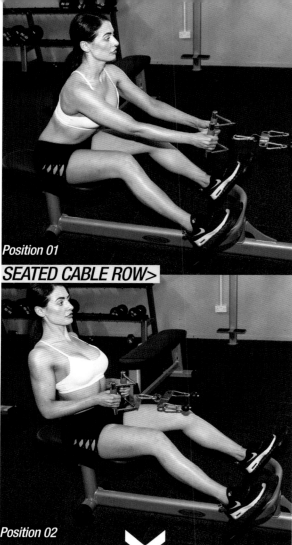

Position 01

SEATED CABLE ROW>

Position 02

> This is a variation on the movement in the wide grip and narrow grip lat pull downs (page 123). For this exercise, you need to attach a V bar to a cable machine. Make sure the seat and weight are adjusted to suit you. Sit into the machine and hold the V bar attachment above your head with your palms facing one another (Position 01). Using the same movement as in the lat pull downs, bring the V bar attachment towards your chest, keeping your arms close to your body (Position 02). Then release and repeat.

> For this exercise you will also use the V bar attachment on the cable machine, but you will need to adjust the chair so that it is low to the ground and about three feet from the tower. Alternatively, you could do it sitting on the floor directly in front of a cable machine. Make sure you set the weight so that it's comfortable for you to lift.

To begin, lean over and grab the handles of the V bar attachment with your palms facing each other. Keep your back nice and strong – don't hunch over (Position 01). As you bring your torso and elbows back, squeeze your shoulder blades together, leaning back slightly to just over 90 degrees (Position 02). Then release your arms forward and repeat.

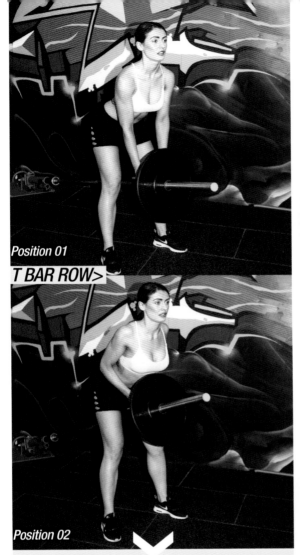

Position 01

T BAR ROW>

Position 02

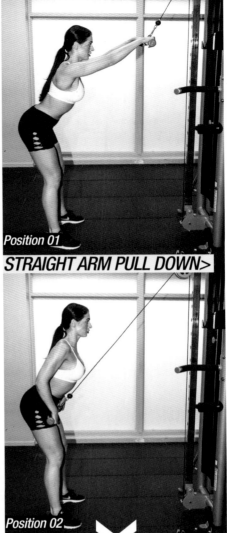

Position 01

STRAIGHT ARM PULL DOWN>

Position 02

> Some gyms have a T bar row machine – if yours does, use it. If not, grab a long bar and insert it into the bar holder or wedged into a corner, just to keep it locked in one place while you complete the exercise. Add the appropriate weight to the free end and stand over the bar, with one leg on either side. With your knees slightly bent, lean your torso forward and grasp the bar below the weights (Position 01). You could use a V bar attachment for easier grip if you want. Begin to bring the bar towards your body, using your elbows and squeezing your back, until the plate tips your body (Position 02). When lowering the bar back down, don't allow it to touch the floor, then repeat.

> Attach a wide bar to a cable machine and set the weight to something you feel comfortable with. Stand directly in front of the tower with your feet wider than shoulder width apart, holding the bar above your head. Your torso should be bent forward slightly (Position 01). Make sure you have enough space between the tower and your body to extend your arms fully. Grip the bar and drive down, using your lats, until the bar reaches your body (Position 02). Then slowly return to Position 01 and repeat.

CARDIO TRAINING

LOW-INTENSITY STEADY STATE EXERCISE (LISS)

LISS refers to steady cardio that can be maintained over a specific period of time. This doesn't mean easy or slow, it means a steady pace that you can keep up over a period of 40–60 minutes.

Try the following activities:

- Steady jogging
- Any of the gym machines, from the bike to the cross trainer
- Walking
- Cycling at a steady speed
- Swimming
- Yoga

HIGH-INTENSITY TRAINING (HIT)

HIT means high-intensity training that is usually done in short bursts and without any rest. This is a great option for anyone looking for a quick, efficient way to exercise. It's also really great at torching body fat and improving muscle condition.

Here are some good HIT options:

- Sprints
- High-intensity plyometrics
- High-intensity circuits
- Weightlifting HIT

HIGH-INTENSITY INTERVAL TRAINING (HIIT)

HIIT is similar to HIT except that is means short, intense bursts followed immediately by a resting period. An example would be sprinting for two minutes, then resting for one minute. There is a range of options to play with. HIIT is a great way to build endurance and speed and it's insanely good for torching body fat. And unlike other forms of cardio, HIIT is also a great way to build and maintain muscle.

Here are some options:

- Sprint and rest
- Battle ropes and rest
- Slam ball and rest

PLYOMETRICS>

Another name for plyometrics is jump training, and it literally means jumping. Plyometrics is a fun way to get fit and I highly recommend adding it to your routine. It's a great way to build power and speed, and it actually helps overall performance across the board.

Here are some brilliant plyo exercises for you to try.>>

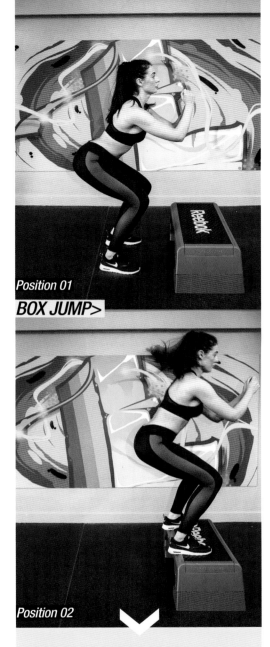

Position 01

BOX JUMP>

Position 02

> For this exercise, you'll need either a step or a box directly in front of you. Start in a standing position, feet hips width part and toes pointing forward. Lower yourself into a squat (Position 01). Jump forward onto the step, trying to jump as high as possible. Land with your knees bent (Position 02). Then step or jump back down and repeat.

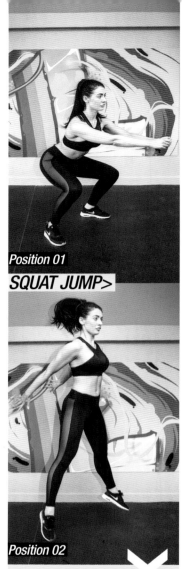

Position 01

SQUAT JUMP>

Position 02

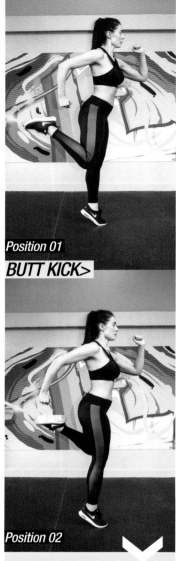

Position 01

BUTT KICK>

Position 02

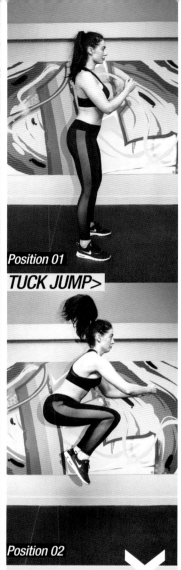

Position 01

TUCK JUMP>

Position 02

> Start in a standing position, feet in a wide stance and toes pointing forward. Lower yourself into a wide squat, with your torso upright and your hands out directly in front of you (Position 01). Jump straight up into the air, bringing your arms behind your body and using your legs to spring up (Position 2). Land and repeat.

> Stand upright with your feet roughly shoulder width apart. Kick your right leg to your bum, swinging your left arm forward (Position 01). Then continue, jumping onto your left leg and swinging your right arm forward (Position 02). Go through the motion almost as if you were running and try to bring each heel as high as possible.

> Start standing upright, with your feet roughly shoulder width apart. Keep your arms out in front of your chest (Position 01). Bring your body down into a high squat to create some force, then jump directly into the air, bringing your knees up towards your chest area (Position 02). Land and repeat, trying to get your knees as high as possible. Be sure to bend your knees as you return to the ground to prevent any ankle injuries.

RESISTANCE TRAINING>

When we talk about resistance training, we mean training that uses resistance to put strain on the muscle. Technically, weight training is included and all forms of weight and resistance training support muscle growth. Weightlifting uses free weights or machines, whereas resistance training uses cables, bands, loops or even your own body weight are hugely beneficial and you should use both for body improvements and overall health.

Here are some upper and lower body exercises using resistance equipment.>>

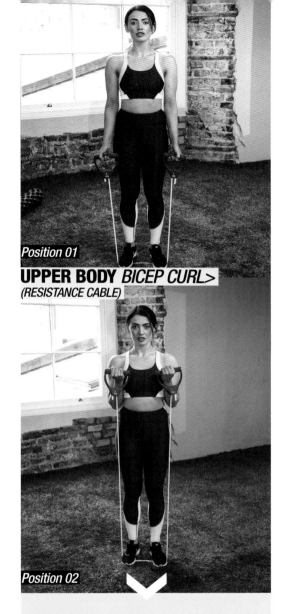

Position 01

UPPER BODY *BICEP CURL>*
(RESISTANCE CABLE)

Position 02

> As with the standard bicep curl (page 109), start by standing upright with your feet hip width apart and your core engaged. Place your resistance cable underneath your feet and hold a handle in each hand, palms towards the body (Position 01). Raise both arms towards your shoulders, contracting your bicep (Position 02). Then lower and repeat.

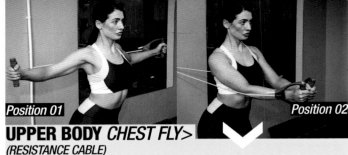

Position 01

Position 02

UPPER BODY CHEST FLY>
(RESISTANCE CABLE)

> This is similar to the cable chest fly (page 119), but uses a resistance cable instead of the cable machine. Before you begin, you'll need to find somewhere clever to loop your resistance cable – perhaps a machine in your gym or a pillar in your house. Position the level of the cable to the middle of your back. Facing away from the cable, grip a handle in each hand with your palms. Leaning slightly forward, extend your arms fully to your sides (Position 01). Then pull the cable towards the front of your body until your hands meet (Position 02). Release and repeat.

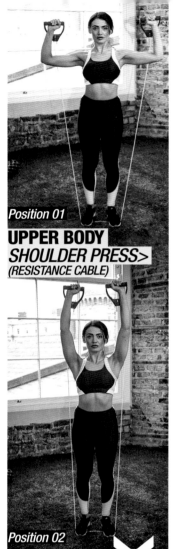

Position 01

UPPER BODY
SHOULDER PRESS>
(RESISTANCE CABLE)

Position 02

> This is a resistance version of the standard shoulder press (page 116). Start standing tall with your feet shoulder width apart and the resistance cable securely underneath your feet. Hold a handle in each hand, with palms facing away from the body. Begin with your arms bent and the handles in line with your head (Position 01). Then push the cables towards the ceiling, extending your arms upwards (Position 02). Bend your arms again and repeat.

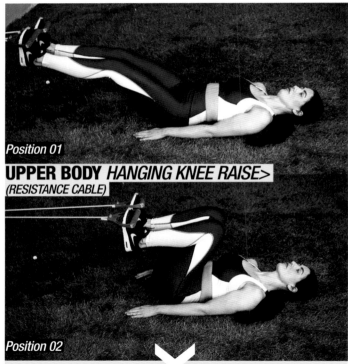

Position 01

UPPER BODY HANGING KNEE RAISE>
(RESISTANCE CABLE)

Position 02

> Again, you will need to find somewhere clever to loop your resistance cable for this exercise. With your back on a mat, hook your feet into the handles of the cable, with your legs extended fully and roughly 45 degrees from the ground (Position 01). Bring both knees towards your body, keeping your legs together. Your calves should be parallel to the floor (Position 02). Then straighten your legs and repeat.

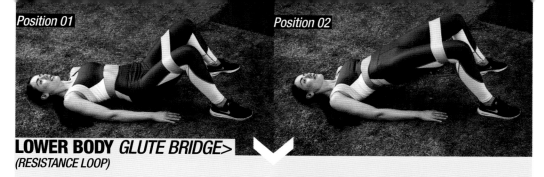

Position 01   Position 02

LOWER BODY *GLUTE BRIDGE>*
(RESISTANCE LOOP)

> This is a variation on the glute bridge on page 94. Start with your back flat on a mat and your legs bent in front of you, with your feet flat on the ground and shoulder width apart. Place your resistance loop around your lower quads, just above the knees (Position 01). Then raise your hips by squeezing your glutes, pausing at the top (Position 02), before lowering down and repeating the movement.

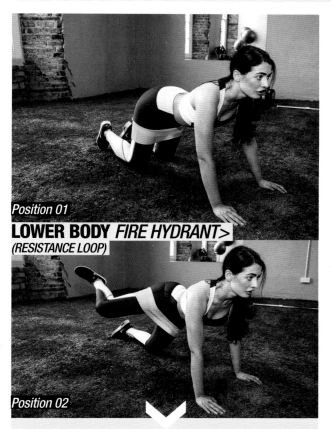

Position 01

LOWER BODY *FIRE HYDRANT>*
(RESISTANCE LOOP)

Position 02

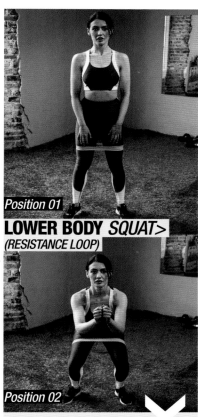

Position 01

LOWER BODY *SQUAT>*
(RESISTANCE LOOP)

Position 02

> Place your resistance loop around your quads and kneel on all fours, with your hands in front of you and your legs hip distance apart (Position 01). Lift your right leg out, keeping the knee bent (Position 02). Then return your leg to the ground and repeat on the left side. Try it without the band first.

> This is a resistance version of the squat on page 92. Start with your feet roughly hip width apart, with the resistance loop around your quads (Position 01). Next, lower yourself, bending your knees and keeping your torso straight, getting as low as you can (Position 02). Push back up to standing and repeat.

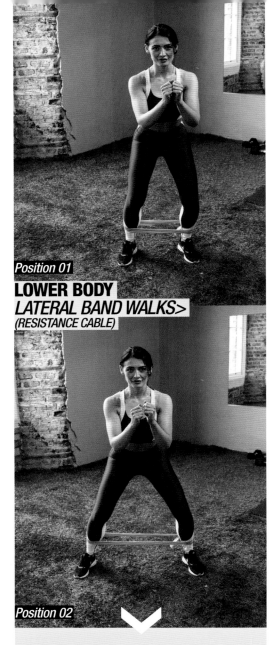

LOWER BODY
LATERAL BAND WALKS>
(RESISTANCE CABLE)

> Start in a squat position with an exercise band or loop around your ankles (Position 01). Keeping your body as low as possible, walk sideways, stepping your leg all the way out to the right (Position 02). Keeping your legs far apart at all times, continue the exercise walking left.

HOW TO READ AN EXERCISE PLAN

Exercise plans can sometimes look overwhelming, but they are really simple and are a great way to stay on track. An exercise plan will typically include goals for one day (leg day, arm day, cardio, etc.). Your plan will start with a warm-up and then move on to the list of exercises you must do, followed by the number of times you need to do each exercise.

When you're just starting out, don't overcomplicate your plan. Take one exercise at a time. If you find yourself a little confused, ask your gym instructor for help. They are there to support the members and would only be delighted to share their wisdom with you.

SETS AND REPS

Sets and reps is the term used to describe the number of times you perform an exercise. A rep (repetition) is the number of times you perform a specific exercise. A set is the number of cycles of reps that you complete.

For example, 'squats 4 x 6' or '4 sets 6 reps 25kg' means the exercise you will do is a squat and you will lift 25kg. You will complete six repetitions of the squat in four cycles, with a break between each cycle. In this example, you would do a total of 24 squats.

Your sets, reps and weight will be based on your goals, whether it's muscle gain, fat loss or toning. It will also depend on your capabilities, i.e. whether you're a novice or more experienced.

Let's look at an example of a typical leg day. Option 1 and Option 2 will give you different results. You will see that Option 1 has fewer repetitions, meaning the focus is on muscle gain and strength, while Option 2 has more repetitions, meaning the focus is on conditioning and toning.

OPTION 1
Lunge 4 x 10
Squat 4 x 8
Leg press 3 x 8
Leg extension 3 x 10
Lying leg curl 3 x 8
Calf raise 3 x 6

OPTION 2
Lunge 4 x 20
Squat 3 x 15
Leg press 3 x 15
Leg extension 3 x 10
Lying leg curl 3 x 10
Calf raise 4 x 15

I made a point of not including a suggested weight in the *BYOB* plans, as the weight is determined by a lot of factors. All beginners should start light and learn how to implement perfect technique, then build the weight up over time as your confidence and your understanding of your body increase. If you're looking to build muscle, the goal is to lift as heavy as possible, but again using perfect technique.

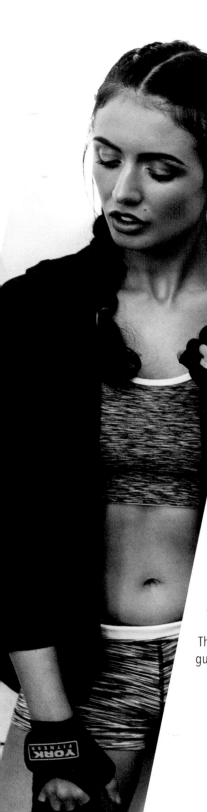

REST AND RECOVERY (R&R)

We have already discussed rest and recovery in other sections throughout *BYOB*, so by now you should know how important they are for improvements and repair and that recovery doesn't mean chilling out on the couch. It refers to the full wheel of optimal recovery, including nutrition, rest, supplements, hydration and stress management. By including R&R as a fundamental part of your cycle, the National Heart, Lung and Blood Institute in the US and the Irish Sports Council say you can maximise your results as well as reset your hormones, improve your mental health and repair your nervous system.

A NOTE ON THE PLANS

Now that you've got some basic moves down, I'll walk you through several different plans designed for different goals:

- *THE TOTAL NEWBIE*
- *TAKE IT TO THE NEXT LEVEL*
- *CURVE NATION*
- *THE BOOTY BUILDER*
- *TONE THAT BOD*
- *SIX PACK DREAMIN'*
- *HEALTHY MIND*
- *THE LONG-TERMER*
- *HOLIDAY EMERGENCY*

The plans aren't written in stone – they're meant to be flexible guidelines that you should adjust to suit your schedule.

A PLAN FOR THE TOTAL NEWBIE

A PLAN FOR THE FITNESS BEGINNER

This plan is designed to get you in the mood for working out, so have fun with it and experiment with each body part. Try this out for three or four weeks as you get to know your body and build some confidence at the gym. Of course, the more active you are, the better, so on your rest days why not go for a walk with one of your best friends or your dog? And as always, be sure to drink plenty of water and take in enough fuel to support your new fitness plan.

MON	TUES	WED	THURS	FRI	SAT	SUN
LOWER BODY	REST	UPPER BODY	REST	CARDIO	LOWER BODY	REST
5–10 min warm-up		5–10 min warm-up		45 mins of LISS exercise (see page 126 for ideas)	5–10 min warm-up	
Leg press 3 x 15		Tricep dip 3 x 15			Leg press 3 x 15	
Leg extension 3 x 15		Bicep curl 4 x 10			Leg extension 3 x 15	
Lying leg curl 4 x 10		Shoulder press 4 x 10			Lying leg curl 4 x 10	
Calf raise 3 x 15		Seated cable row 3 x 15			Calf raise 3 x 15	
Donkey kick 4 x 10		Incline chest press 3 x 10			Donkey kick 4 x 10	
Butt kick 20 reps		Crunch 3 x 20			Butt kick 20 reps	

TAKE IT TO THE NEXT LEVEL

A PLAN FOR THE GIRL WHO WANTS TO TAKE IT TO NEXT STAGE

This plan is designed for the more experienced lady who is ready to train each body part as well as make some progress with fat loss.

MON	TUES	WED	THURS	FRI	SAT	SUN
QUADS AND CALVES	REST	CHEST, SHOULDERS AND BACK	REST	CARDIO AND ABS	GLUTES AND HAMSTRINGS	REST
5–10 min warm-up		5–10 min warm-up		5–10 min warm-up	5–10 min warm-up	
Lunge 4 x 10		Lateral raise 3 x 15		20 min HIIT: 3 min as fast as possible, rest until you feel recovered, then continue.	Glute bridge 3 x 10	
Squat 3 x 10		Barbell military press 3 x 15		V sit-up with stability ball 3 x 20	Squat 3 x 10	
Leg press 4 x 10		Cable chest fly 4 x 10		Hanging knee raise 3 x 15	Donkey kick 4 x 15	
Narrow stance squat 4 x 10		Bent over row 3 x 10		Side plank 4 x 60 secs	Good morning 4 x 15	
Calf raise 3 x 15		V bar pull down 3 x 15			Lying leg curl 4 x 15	
Leg extension 3 x 15		Incline chest press 3 x 10			Box jump 4 x 20	

CURVE NATION

FOR THE GIRL WHO WANTS TO GROW SOME SEXY MUSCLES ALL OVER

This is a workout plan for a lady with some experience, so it's not suitable for beginners. If you're a total novice, you can try this plan once you are comfortable in a gym environment and most importantly, once you have nailed the technique with lighter weights.

This is a great workout plan for the lady who is serious about training and wants to build muscle from head to toe. Try it for a six- to eight-week period. Remember, it's impossible to grow muscle without sustenance, so make sure you're eating enough to support intense workouts, repair and growth. Eat big to get big!

You will also notice that there is no cardio in this plan, as the main goal is to grow. You must try to lift as heavy as possible in this plan, with fewer repetitions – really challenge yourself.

MON	TUES	WED	THURS	FRI	SAT	SUN
QUADS AND CALVES	**CHEST**	**BACK**	**GLUTES AND HAMSTRINGS**	**REST**	**SHOULDERS AND ABS**	**REST**
5–10 min warm-up	5–10 min warm-up	5–10 min warm-up	5–10 min warm-up		5–10 min warm-up	
Lunge 4 x 6	Cable chest fly (using lighter weights) 4 x 15	T bar row 4 x 6	Glute bridge 4 x 6		Shoulder press 4 x 8	
Squat 4 x 8	Incline chest press 4 x 6	Wide grip lat pull down 3 x 10	Squat 4 x 6		Lateral raise 4 x 8	
Leg press 4 x 8	Bench press 4 x 8	Narrow grip lat pull down 3 x 10	Donkey kick 4 x 15		Rear delt fly 4 x 8	
Leg extension 4 x 8	Cable chest fly (using lighter weights) 4 x 15	Bent over row 3 x 6	Lying leg curl 4 x 8		Upright row 3 x 10	
Calf raise 4 x 8	Bench press 4 x 6	V bar pull down 4 x 8	Bulgarian split squat 3 x 6		Medicine ball twist 4 x 10	
Leg press using a smith machine 4 x 8		Seated cable row 3 x 10	Cable pull through 3 x 10		Hanging knee raise 4 x 10	

THE BOOTY BUILDER
FOR THE LADY LOOKING TO BUILD THAT BUM

Building a great booty takes time and commitment. In this plan the glutes are the focus – you will see that they are targeted three times a week. Technique is so important for this plan, as using the perfect technique means engaging the muscles and making them work. Perfect your technique using lighter weights before lifting heavy. Build yourself up to heavier weights in the previous plans and get comfortable and confident, as building a serious booty takes a little more experience. You should feel each exercise working the glutes significantly, and that can sometimes mean thinking about the area and focusing on it.

If you find that your glutes are a difficult area to work with, try pre-exhausting them using a resistance loop:

• Fire hydrant using a resistance loop 4 x 25
• Glute bridges using a resistance loop 4 x 25

Also remember to fuel up and eat right, as building a dream booty takes a serious amount of energy. And as always, aid your recovery with supplements and rest.

MON	TUES	WED	THURS	FRI	SAT	SUN
QUADS AND GLUTES	REST	BACK, CHEST AND SHOULDERS	GLUTES AND HAMSTRINGS	REST	GLUTES AND ABS	REST
5–10 min warm-up		5–10 min warm-up	5–10 min warm-up		5–10 min warm-up	
Lunge 4 x 6		Lateral raise 4 x 10	Glute bridge 3 x 10		Sumo squat 4 x 8	
Squat 4 x 8		Bench press 3 x 8	Squat 3 x 10		Kickback on a smith machine 4 x 10	
Leg press 4 x 8		Shoulder press 3 x 8	Donkey kick 4 x 15		Glute bridge 4 x 8	
Leg extension 4 x 8		Bent over row 3 x 10	Lying leg curl 4 x 8		Cable pull through 4 x 10	
Calf raise 4 x 8		V bar pull down 3 x 15	Kickback on a smith machine 4 x 10		V sit-up with a stability ball 4 x 20	
Glute bridge 3 x 10		Cable chest fly 4 x 10	Step-up 4 x 15		Hanging knee raise 4 x 20	

TONE THAT BOD

FOR THE LADY WHO WANTS TO TONE HER BOD FROM TOP TO TOE

This plan is focused on full-body toning, which includes more resistance training, plyometrics and high reps. If you're looking to tighten everything up, then this is the plan for you. This is also a great one for beginners who are ready for a more difficult plan, as it's a lot of fun and utilises lighter weights, meaning you have a chance to familiarise yourself with your form and technique and build your confidence.

MON	TUES	WED	THURS	FRI	SAT	SUN
UPPER BODY AND CARDIO	**LOWER BODY**	**UPPER BODY AND CARDIO**	**LOWER BODY**	**PLYO AND CORE**	**REST**	**REST**
5–10 min warm-up	5–10 min warm-up	5–10 min warm-up	5–10 min warm-up	5–10 min warm-up		
Tricep dip 4 x 15	Box jump 4 x 20	HIIT for 2 mins, then recover – repeat for 20 min	Glute bridge (resistance loop) 4 x 15	Tuck jump 4 x 20		
Bicep curl (resistance cable) 4 x 15	Squat (resistance loop) 4 x 15	Tricep dip 4 x 15	Squat 3 x 15	Push-up 4 x 20		
Shoulder press (resistance cable) 4 x 15	Leg press 4 x 15	Lateral raise 4 x 15	Fire hydrant 4 x 15	Squat jump 4 x 20		
Cable chest fly 4 x 15	Glute bridge 4 x 15	Bicep curl (resistance cable) 4 x 15	Lying leg curl 4 x 15	Plank 4 x 60 secs		
Lateral raise 4 x 18	Step-up 4 x 20	Incline chest press 4 x 15	Lunge 4 x 20	Toe toucher 4 x 25		
HIIT cardio for 10 mins: 60 secs on, 60 secs rest	Fire hydrant 4 x 15	Seated cable row 4 x 15	25 min of LISS cardio	TRX crunch 4 x 10		

SIX PACK DREAMIN'

BUILD THE STOMACH OF YOUR DREAMS

Now that you know all about your abs, you know the importance of a healthy diet for dropping body fat around the stomach area. That being said, it's also important to build core strength and work on those ab and oblique developments. This plan is focused on dropping fat and showcasing those rock-hard abductors. Drink plenty of water, eat loads of green vegetables and stick to a consistent diet plan to maximise results.

MON	TUES	WED	THURS	FRI	SAT	SUN
CARDIO AND ABS	**LOWER BODY**	**UPPER BODY**	**CARDIO AND ABS**	**REST**	**CARDIO AND ABS**	**REST**
5–10 min warm-up	5–10 min warm-up	5–10 min warm-up	5–10 min warm-up		5–10 min warm-up	
HIIT: 2 min on, then recover – repeat for 20 mins	Leg press 4 x 15	Barbell military press 4 x 15	HIIT: 2 min on, then recover – repeat for 20 mins		HIIT: 2 min on, then recover – repeat for 20 mins	
TRX crunch 4 x 10	Leg extension 4 x 10	Incline chest press 4 x 10	Toe toucher 4 x 15		Crunch 4 x 15	
Plank 3 x 10	Curtsy squat 4 x 10	Skull crusher 4 x 15	TRX crunch 4 x 10		Hanging knee raise 3 x 10	
V sit-up with stability ball 4 x 10	Calf raise 4 x 15	Bent over row 3 x 10	Hanging knee raise 3 x 10		Side plank 4 x 15	
Medicine ball twist 4 x 15	Lying leg curl 4 x 10	V bar pull down 3 x 15	Side plank 4 x 60 secs		TRX crunch 4 x 10	
Crunch 4 x 15	Glute bridge 4 x 10	Bicep curl 4 x 15	Medicine ball slam 4 x 10		Plank 4 x 60 secs	

HEALTHY MIND

EXERCISE YOUR WAY TO A HAPPY, HEALTHY MIND

I really wanted to include a plan like this for the person who is lacking motivation and is basically not feeling 100% themselves. With this plan, the most important thing is to just get moving every day. As you know, exercise improves mood, so give it a shot, even just for one week, and I promise you'll feel better. This plan isn't focused on performance or aesthetics, but rather on having a feel-good week. When I felt low in the past, going for a walk with my dog for 30 minutes a day made a significant change in my mood and I found myself with more clarity and peace.

This plan is pretty simple and uncomplicated, but if you're feeling more adventurous, try going to a class at your local gym instead of walking. The most important thing is to just do something.

MON	TUES	WED	THURS	FRI	SAT	SUN
RELAXED CARDIO	RELAXED CARDIO	BODY AND MIND	RELAXED CARDIO	BODY AND MIND	RELAXED CARDIO	OUTDOORS
30 min walking outside	30 min walking outside	Pilates or yoga class	30 min walking outside	Pilates or yoga class	30 min walking outside	2 hr hill walk *(take advantage of your local mountains)*

THE LONG-TERMER

FOR THE GIRL WHO WANTS A CONSISTENT PLAN

Welcome to the long-term plan for the fitness goddess who realises the importance of consistency and who wants this to become part of her life for the long haul. This plan is a mix of aspects from the above plans, with a combination of cardio, mental happiness, weight training and plyometrics. As your knowledge grows, you can be more experimental and you will also know the areas you need to focus on and challenge. Remember, face your weaknesses head on and improve them.

MON	TUES	WED	THURS	FRI	SAT	SUN
CHEST, BACK AND CARDIO	QUADS, GLUTES AND HAMSTRINGS	CARDIO	BICEPS, TRICEPS AND SHOULDERS	ABS, CARDIO AND PLYOS	REST	REST
5–10 min warm-up	5–10 min warm-up	5–10 min warm-up	5–10 min warm-up	5–10 min warm-up		
Bent over row 3 x 10	Sumo squat 4 x 8	45 min of LISS	Tricep rope pull down 3 x 15	HIIT: 2 min on, 1 min rest – repeat for 20 mins		
Incline chest press 3 x 10	Lunge 4 x 10		Barbell military press 4 x 10	Box jump 4 x 20		
Wide grip lat pull down 4 x 10	Calf raise 4 x 15		Bicep curl 4 x 10	TRX crunch 4 x 15		
V bar pull down 3 x 15	Glute bridge 4 x 10		Rear delt fly 4 x 10	V sit-up with a stability ball 3 x 15		
Bench press 3 x 15	Donkey kick 3 x 15		Skull crusher 3 x 15	TRX oblique crunch 4 x 15		
Cable chest fly 4 x 10	Lying leg curl 3 x 10		Barbell curl 4 x 10	Tuck jump 4 x 15		
10 min of HIIT: 60 secs on, 30 secs rest	Leg press 3 x 10		Upright row 4 x 10	Ab knee raise (resistance cable) 4 x 15		
	Narrow stance squat 4 x 10					

HOLIDAY EMERGENCY

SIX-WEEK EMERGENCY PLAN TO LOOK AND FEEL GREAT

We've all been there – your holiday is creeping up and you're not ready to stick on that bikini. I am totally against short-term quick fixes because we all know about relapses and rebounds, so look at this as a six-week introduction to health instead. It should be immediately followed with one of the other plans with the goal of maintaining health and fitness in the long term.

This plan incorporates a lot of resistance and conditioning-style training to help you look your best on the beach and in your holiday photos. When using higher reps, remember to keep your weight manageable so that you can complete every rep.

MON	TUES	WED	THURS	FRI	SAT	SUN
FULL-BODY BLAST	**CARDIO AND GLUTES**	**FULL-BODY BLAST**	**ABS AND CARDIO**	**REST**	**FULL-BODY BLAST**	**CARDIO**
5–10 min warm-up	5–10 min warm-up	5–10 min warm-up	5–10 min warm-up		5–10 min warm-up	5–10 min warm-up
Lunge 4 x 20	Glute bridge 4 x 10	Push-up 4 x 20	20 mins of HIIT		Squat 4 x 20	60 mins of LISS
Push-up 4 x 20	Donkey kick 3 x 15	Tricep dip 4 x 15	Plank 4 x 60 secs		Lunge 4 x 20	
Shoulder press 4 x 20	Lateral band walk 4 x 25	Sumo squat 4 x 8	Side plank 4 x 60 secs		Bicep curl *(resistance cable)* 4 x 15	
Hammer curl 3 x 15	Kickback on a smith machine 3 x 15	Barbell curl 4 x 15	Scissors 4 x 10		Calf raise 4 x 15	
Curtsy squat 3 x 15	Cable pull through 4 x 15	Leg extension 4 x 15	TRX crunch 3 x 15		Bench press 4 x 15	
Cable chest fly 3 x 10	Reverse hyperextension 4 x 10	Tuck jump 4 x 20	TRX oblique crunch 3 x 15		Good morning 4 x 15	
Leg press 4 x 15	10 min of HIT	Narrow grip lat pull down 4 x 10	Medicine ball slam 4 x 20		Reverse hyperextension 4 x 10	

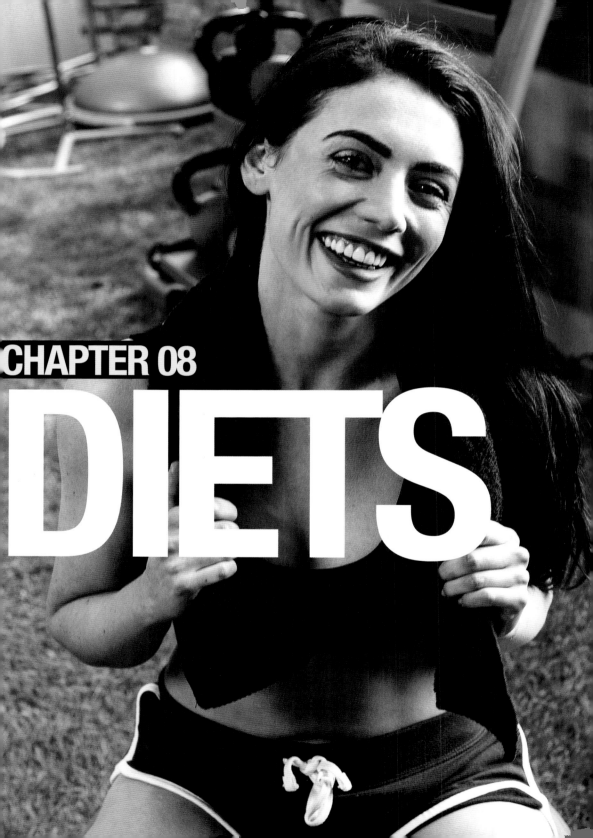

CHAPTER 08
DIETS

Much like the workout plans in the previous chapter, in this chapter I'll give you some ideas for diet plans designed for different goals. I'll also introduce you to the theory behind functional eating as well as carb cycling and carb manipulation.

But first, we'll talk about what a good diet plan can do for you, how to use cheat meals and rewards, and how to figure out your calorie needs, resting metabolic rate and macro needs. I've also included the nutritional values of some of the most common foods you should be eating so that you can have this information at your fingertips.

So many young women still believe that the only way to lose weight is by restricting or starving themselves, but I'm happy to tell you that the *BYOB* diet plans do not buy into that. A healthy relationship with food and even just a basic understanding of nutrition are going to help you kick ass.

DIET PLANS: THE GOOD, THE BAD AND THE UGLY

A good diet plan maintains or improves overall health and well-being. It ensures you have a balanced diet with the right amounts of protein, carbohydrates and fats. Each food group serves an important purpose and you need all three to function at your best.

On the other hand, a diet consisting of takeaways, chocolate, sugary cereal, processed meats and fizzy drinks will not only see your weight increase, but it will see your health diminish too. Studies published in the *Obesity* research journal and *Time* magazine have shown that a bad diet can have a seriously negative impact on the body after as little as five days. Authority Nutrition explains that the ability to oxidise glucose is corrupted, meaning your body can't break down carbohydrates and in turn stores more as fat.

So the first issue with a bad diet is a destroyed metabolism, future carbohydrate resistance and an increase in body fat. Secondly, the World Heart Federation, Harvard Medical School, Irish Health and Diabetes Ireland state that eating a poor diet can cause huge hazards to your health, including a greater risk of disease and illness. Diabetes and heart disease are just two of the dangers of a bad diet.

DIET PLANS ARE NOT ONE-SIZE-FITS-ALL

Every single person is unique and special. Our interests, our hobbies, our learning abilities – you name it, and we are all so different. The exact same thing applies to diet plans and even exercise. It is only in the doing that you can really see what works and what doesn't work for you. At the same time, you can't be expected to know that a particular food or diet plan doesn't work for you after one short week; it takes a little time. After two years of experimenting with theories and plans, I now know what agrees with me and what doesn't, but what works for me won't necessarily work for you.

You'll often see people online and in professional reports state one theory as being fact, and then another person will come along who will argue the exact opposite theory as fact. My theory is that we are all bio-individual and should focus on our own bodies and be body aware. **There are so many options and no one plan is right for everyone.** It's about eating intuitively and seeing the reaction it has on you. It's about monitoring things like how you feel after eating certain foods: do you have more energy or less? Are you bloated? How did it affect your bowel movement? The only one guarantee is that good, healthy food works, but as you develop and improve, you will be able to notice the different impacts that even healthy food has on your body.

A huge part of this theory is down to lifestyle. Some people have physically demanding jobs while others are more sedentary, so both of those people will automatically have different diet needs. If you exercise a lot you will clearly need more calories than somebody who is inactive. In short, the diet plan for J-LO may not be the diet plan for you, but that doesn't mean you can't figure out what your perfect nutrition plan is – one that works with your lifestyle, with your individuality and with your goals in mind. Who wants to be like everybody else anyway?

HOW TO SPICE UP YOUR DIET PLAN

We are the online generation, so if you need some inspiration when it comes to healthy eating, then jump online and follow some of the healthy food enthusiasts who share their healthy recipe ideas and tips. Some of my favourite bloggers are Joe Wicks (The Body Coach), India Power (The Little Green Spoon) and Ella Woodward (Deliciously Ella).

Healthy food doesn't mean boring food! By getting excited and imaginative you can create a colourful, complete, exciting and delicious meal that will not only offer flavour, but an explosion of nutrients too.

Try the following tips:

- Use bright, colourful fruit and vegetables. As the saying goes, 'eat the rainbow' to make sure you're getting the wide range of nutrients your body needs.

- Mix it up! Try to eat different things every day and switch your proteins, carbs and veg. Every day should offer a fresh flavour.

- Try new things. Use this as your opportunity to step outside of the box when it comes to healthy food. For example, I recently tried squid for the first time and now I include it in my diet on a regular basis.

HOW TO USE CHEAT MEALS AND REWARDS

It is totally unrealistic to think that anybody can maintain a diet 24/7 without a little relief now and then. But guess what? **Not only is it 100% possible to indulge in your favourite sweets and enjoy a treat without ruining all of your hard work, but you can even boost fat loss using cheat meals!**

Rewards and cheat meals are a little different. A reward is unscheduled and should be based on the 80/20 rule: you follow a healthy, nutritious diet 80% of the time and you give yourself some leeway for the other 20%. It's a more relaxed way of looking at things that helps you maintain a healthy lifestyle for the long term rather than just in short bursts. On the other hand, a cheat meal is a scheduled treat that usually has more nutritious value – it's mostly high in carbohydrates and protein levels, which help restore lost glycogen levels in the muscle from a tough week of training and eating clean.

Both are only allowed based on efforts and should be seen as compensation, as this type of food is usually low in nutritive value. Both options are a great way to have a healthy and controlled relationship with all foods, even the 'bad' ones. By having treats on a regular basis, you can also prevent yourself from falling into the binge–purge cycle as you can plan for it and look forward to it. The most important thing is to not allow your cheat or reward to run away with you – don't let either one turn into a full day or week of eating junk food. But if you slip up sometimes, who cares? Look at it as a reward that you obviously needed. Just don't take advantage of the system or you could undo all of your hard work. Balance is key.

HOW A CHEAT MEAL CAN HELP WEIGHT LOSS

- Eating a cheat meal once or twice a week can offer both mental and weight loss advantages.

- A cheat meal replenishes glycogen.

- A cheat meal replenishes hormones, which can aid normal metabolism and insulin levels.

- A cheat meal preserves calorie-burning and fat-loss properties.

- A cheat meal offers a motivational incentive to continue with a healthy diet plan.

- A cheat meal offers a controlled way to enjoy treats.

(Sources: Dr Susie Rockway, MedicalDaily.com, *Muscle & Fitness* magazine, Livestrong.com.)

WHY THE 80/20 RULE OFFERS THE GREATEST POTENTIAL FOR A LONG-TERM HEALTHY LIFESTYLE

- It gives you room to enjoy more variety in your daily nutritional plan.

- It's the best option for fitness newbies.

- It's more spontaneous.

- It's a realistic plan and approach to healthy living.

- It gives you a mental break too.

- It allows you to still enjoy a social life.

- It gives you opportunities to enjoy a treat guilt free.

HOW TO DETERMINE YOUR DIET PLAN

To create a diet plan that works for you, you'll first need to figure out your calorie needs and your basal metabolic rate (BMR). I could go into the science behind the Harris Benedict equation, which determines your calorie needs by accounting for your activity requirements along with things like height, weight and age, but suffice it to say that the easiest way to figure it out is to use an online calorie and BMR calculator (try My Fitness Pal, a fantastic app that will help you determine your calorie needs). Your calorie requirements could be anywhere from 1,750 to 2,500 calories or more based on your goals. It might sound like a lot, but remember, you want to eat enough to give you the energy you need to perform in the gym.

The calculator will tell you your BMR, which is the calories you burn during rest. Based on your activity level, it will also tell you how many calories you should be eating each day. By following these guidelines, you can plan your week much more efficiently. Plus this way, you can also avoid undereating or overeating. When you figure out how many calories you need for a day, you can then determine the breakdown. A good starting point according to My Fitness Pal is **20% fat, 30% protein and 50% carbohydrates**. Once you get into a good routine with that format, you can play around with your macronutrient needs. For example, if you are reducing your carbohydrates, you will need to counter that by increasing your protein intake.

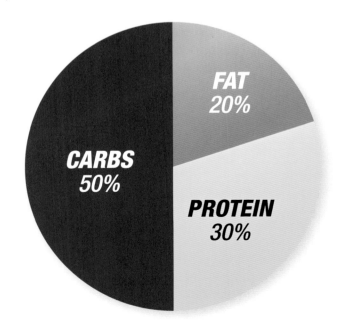

Source: My Fitness Pal

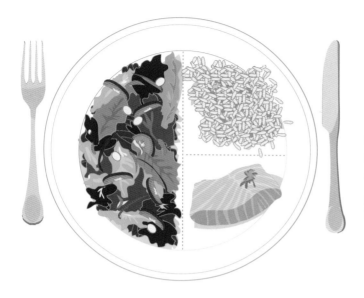

HERE IS WHAT YOUR FOOD PLATE SHOULD LOOK LIKE.

Source: My Fitness Pal recommendation of 20% fat, 30% protein and 50% carbohydrates

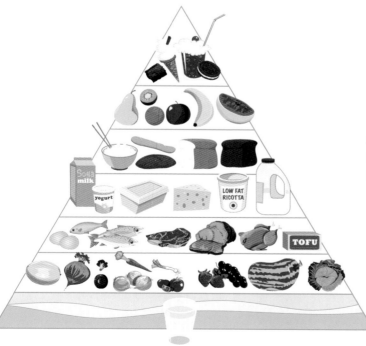

AND HERE'S THE FOOD CHART YOU SHOULD FOLLOW IF YOU WANT TO GET RIPPED.

HYDRATION

You can see that water is a big part of my amended food pyramid. Water is the number one most essential nutrient that the body needs to function, grow and repair. It is so underestimated and undervalued, but it offers huge health benefits. According to the NHS, the Mayo Clinic, Harvard Medical School and Kidney Health Australia, water is a natural hunger suppressant, it removes toxins in the body and it supports the transport of waste. It can improve skin condition and being hydrated helps to avoid fatigue. Most importantly, water transports nutrients throughout your body, be it to your brain or your muscles. Drinking plenty of water also supports fat loss by supporting the kidney functions.

Adults should drink at least 2 litres of water per day to support normal body function and maintain health. Being even slightly dehydrated can have serious health risks. Human Kinetics lists reduced muscle response, strength and co-ordination as a few of the effects of dehydration, while according to Matthew Kempton and Ulrich Ettinger from the Institute of Psychiatry, Psychology and Neuroscience at King's College London, it can even shrink your brain, so drink up, ladies!

NUTRITIONAL VALUES

The following tables show the nutritional values of some of the most common foods that you should be eating, which will make it easier to figure out your needs for the day. I'm not suggesting that you become a slave to calorie counting, because that's not a lifestyle change. Rather, this is just a good source of information to have at your fingertips. **Knowledge is power, and the more you know about the food you're eating, the better.**

VEGETABLES

ARTICHOKES (100G)	47 calories	0.2g fat	11.0g carbs	3.3g protein
ASPARAGUS (100G)	20 calories	0.1g fat	3.9g carbs	2.2g protein
AUBERGINES (100G)	25 calories	0.2g fat	6.0g carbs	1.0g protein
BELL PEPPERS (100G)	20 calories	0.2g fat	4.6g carbs	0.9g protein
BROCCOLI (100G)	34 calories	0.4g fat	7.0g carbs	2.8g protein
BRUSSELS SPROUTS (100G)	43 calories	0.3g fat	9.0g carbs	3.4g protein
CABBAGE (100G)	25 calories	0.1g fat	6.0g carbs	1.3g protein
CARROTS (100G)	41 calories	0.2g fat	10.0g carbs	0.9g protein
CAULIFLOWER (100G)	25 calories	0.3g fat	5.0g carbs	1.9g protein
CELERY (100G)	16 calories	0.2g fat	3.0g carbs	0.7g protein

COURGETTES (100G)	17 calories	0.3g fat	3.1g carbs	1.2g protein
GREEN BEANS (100G)	31 calories	0.1g fat	7.0g carbs	1.8g protein
KALE (100G)	49 calories	0.9g fat	9.0g carbs	4.3g protein
LETTUCE (100G)	15 calories	0.2g fat	2.9g carbs	1.4g protein
MUSHROOMS (100G)	13 calories	0.1g fat	0.1g carbs	0.5g protein
PEAS (100G)	81 calories	0.4g fat	14.0g carbs	5.0g protein
ROCKET (100G)	25 calories	0.7g fat	3.7g carbs	2.6g protein
SPINACH (100G)	23 calories	0.4g fat	3.6g carbs	2.9g protein
TOMATOES (100G)	18 calories	0.2g fat	3.9g carbs	0.9g protein
TURNIPS (100G)	28 calories	0.1g fat	6.0g carbs	0.9g protein

PROTEINS

CHICKEN BREAST, LEAN (170G)	205 calories	4.0g fat	0g carbs	38.0g protein
EGG WHITES (100G)	52 calories	0.2g fat	0.7g carbs	11.0g protein
EGGS (100G)	155 calories	11.0g fat	1.1g carbs	13.0g protein
LEAN ROUND STEAK (115G)	138 calories	4.0g fat	0g carbs	24.0g protein
PRAWNS (100G)	105 calories	1.7g fat	0.9g carbs	20.0g protein
SALMON FILLET, LEAN (115G)	208 calories	12.0g fat	0g carbs	23.0g protein
SQUID (28G)	70 calories	0g fat	0g carbs	15.0g protein
TIN OF TUNA IN BRINE (120G)	150 calories	0g fat	0g carbs	35.0g protein
TUNA STEAK (100G)	107 calories	1.0g fat	0g carbs	25.0g protein
TURKEY (100G LEAN TURKEY, NO SKIN)	135 calories	1g fat	0g carbs	30.0g protein
WHITE FISH, BAKED (100G)	52 calories	0g fat	0g carbs	12.0g protein

CARBOHYDRATES

BROWN BREAD (50G)	98 calories	0.8g fat	22.0g carbs	3.0g protein
BROWN PASTA (100G)	255 calories	2.0g fat	49.0g carbs	11.0g protein
BROWN RICE (1 CUP)	215 calories	3.0g fat	45.0g carbs	5.0g protein
BUTTER BEANS (100G)	115 calories	0.4g fat	21.0g carbs	8.0g protein
CHICKPEAS (100G)	364 calories	6.0g fat	61.0g carbs	19.0g protein
COUSCOUS (1 CUP)	176 calories	0.3g fat	37.0g carbs	6.0g protein
LENTILS (100G)	116 calories	0.4g fat	20.0g carbs	9.0g protein
OATS (40G)	150 calories	2.0g fat	29.0g carbs	4.0g protein

SWEET POTATOES (100G)	86 calories	0g fat	20.0g carbs	1.6g protein
WHITE POTATOES (100G)	86 calories	0g fat	19.4g carbs	2.0g protein
WHITE RICE (1 CUP)	204 calories	0.4g fat	44.0g carbs	4.0g protein

FATS

ALMOND BUTTER (1 TBSP)	102 calories	9.0g fat	2.8g carbs	3.4g protein
ALMONDS (40G)	230 calories	19.6g fat	8.8g carbs	8.4g protein
AVOCADO (100G)	160 calories	15.0g fat	9.0g carbs	2.0g protein
CASHEW BUTTER (1 TBSP)	94 calories	7.9g fat	4.4g carbs	2.8g protein
CASHEWS (40G)	221 calories	17.6g fat	12.0g carbs	7.2g protein
CHIA SEEDS (16G)	60 calories	3.0g fat	5.0g carbs	3.0g protein
COCONUT OIL (1 TBSP)	117 calories	13.6g fat	0g carbs	0g protein
FLAXSEEDS (32G)	60 calories	5.0g fat	4.0g carbs	3.0g protein
HAZELNUTS (40G)	251 calories	24.4g fat	6.8g carbs	6.0g protein
OLIVE OIL (1 TBSP)	119 calories	13.5g fat	0g carbs	0g protein
PEANUT BUTTER (1 TBSP)	94 calories	8.0g fat	3.0g carbs	4.0g protein
PEANUTS (40G)	227 calories	19.6g fat	6.4g carbs	10.4g protein
PECANS (40G)	276 calories	28.8g fat	5.6g carbs	3.6g protein
PISTACHIOS (40G)	225 calories	18.0g fat	11.2g carbs	8.0g protein
WALNUTS (40G)	262 calories	26.0g fat	5.6g carbs	6.0g protein

FRUIT

APPLE (100G)	52 calories	0.2g fat	14.0g carbs	0.3g protein
BANANA (100G)	89 calories	0.3g fat	23.0g carbs	1.1g protein
BLUEBERRIES (100G)	57 calories	0.3g fat	14.0g carbs	0.7g protein
GRAPEFRUIT (100G)	42 calories	0.1g fat	11.0g carbs	0.8g protein
GRAPES (100G)	67 calories	0.4g fat	17.0g carbs	0.6g protein
KIWI (100G)	61 calories	0.5g fat	15.0g carbs	1.1g protein
LEMON (100G)	29 calories	0.3g fat	9.0g carbs	1.1g protein
LIME (100G)	30 calories	0.2g fat	11.0g carbs	0.7g protein
MANGO (100G)	60 calories	0.8g fat	15.0g carbs	0.8g protein
MELON (100G)	28 calories	0.1g fat	7.0g carbs	1.1g protein
ORANGE (100G)	47 calories	0.1g fat	12.0g carbs	0.9g protein
PEACH (100G)	39 calories	0.3g fat	10.0g carbs	0.9g protein

PEAR (100G)	57 calories	0.1g fat	15.0g carbs	0.4g protein
PINEAPPLE (100G)	120 calories	4.0g fat	21.0g carbs	1.0g protein
RASPBERRIES (100G)	53 calories	0.7g fat	12.0g carbs	1.2g protein
STRAWBERRIES (100G)	33 calories	0.3g fat	8.0g carbs	0.7g protein

TREATS

DARK CHOCOLATE (100G)	580 calories	42.0g fat	36.5g carbs	9.1g protein
GREEK YOGURT (100G)	59 calories	0.4g fat	3.6g carbs	10.0g protein
HONEY (50G)	152 calories	0g fat	41.0g carbs	0.1g protein

(Source: My Fitness Pal)

WHAT *NOT* TO EAT

You should avoid the following treats as much as possible unless they're a reward or part of a controlled cheat meal:

- Cakes, sugar and sweets
- Carbonated drinks
- Cereal
- Crisps
- Diet foods and drinks
- Fried foods
- Pre-made and packaged juices and smoothies
- Processed junk food
- Processed meats
- Sugar
- Takeaway foods
- White bread and pasta

SMOKING AND ALCOHOL

Cheat meals and rewards are fine, but cigarettes and alcohol are not. **There are no two ways about it: smoking and drinking alcohol are off limits if you're determined to make physical, mental and athletic improvements.** Fitness is about health from the inside out, and smoking and alcohol are two toxins that are not going to do you, your fitness goals or your long-term health any favours.

Smoking cigarettes can cause an increase in heart rate, blood pressure and hormone production and it can even affect your metabolism. When you smoke, you're taking in over 4,000 chemicals that are destined to cause heart disease, hazardous blood circulation problems and a range of other illnesses. You also speed up the ageing process and limit your fitness results due to a lack of oxygen in your body, which is needed for repair and growth.

Alcohol is a no-no too. Alcohol affects the body in many negative ways, including reduced blood flow around the body, which is essential for maintaining healthy muscles. It also affects your energy levels and reduces your blood sugar level.

Alcohol is high in calories but empty on nutrition. It offers no value whatsoever.

If you enjoy a couple of drinks, do so once every six to eight weeks. Don't throw away all your hard work by getting trapped in a cycle of binge drinking every weekend. The same goes for smoking too. Save all the money you'd spend on cigarettes and spend it on something that has a positive impact on your life instead, like a holiday.

(Sources: American Lung Association, HSE, Irish Cancer Society, Irish Heart Foundation, *Journal of the American College of Cardiology, Muscles, Ligaments and Tendons Journal* and Quit.ie.)

A NOTE ON THE PLANS

These plans are just guidelines and are meant to give you some inspiration. A diet plan should work with you and your lifestyle. You should always consult your GP, a nutritionist or a professional dietician for more detailed nutrition advice, but having said that, here are a few other things to take into account – and be sure to use the templates on pages 190–192 to create your own diet plans.

DON'T FORGET YOUR CALORIE INTAKE

I haven't accounted for calorie or macro needs in these diet plans, as I can't tell each and every one of you what your needs are. But the good news is that it's easy to figure it out using an online calorie counter to design a plan that's perfect for you.

BE BODY CONSCIOUS

Some foods will work for you and some won't. Be aware of changes like bloating or heartburn. If a particular food doesn't agree with you, change it for one that does.

EAT WHAT YOU FANCY

I hate mushrooms, but that doesn't mean that *you* shouldn't eat mushrooms! Switch things up to suit your own personal tastes.

CHOOSE YOUR FOODS WISELY

Don't forget to read the list on pages 150–153 of some of the foods that you should be eating – as well as the foods that you *shouldn't* be eating. Use that information to help plan your meals.

WATER

Don't forget to drink plenty of water – seriously, it will do wonders for you. Try to drink at least 2 litres a day. I usually drink 2 litres just during my workout.

SUPPLEMENTS

Your supplement plan should be based on your goals, whether it's muscle growth or fat loss. Start simple with vitamins, minerals and a protein shake. Read Chapter 5 for more information about supplements.

ENJOY IT!

Lastly, be sure you enjoy your meals. Good, healthy food is delicious.

THE BALANCE PLAN

A plan for both the newbie and the long-term girl who wants to make fitness a lifetime relationship

When you adopt the fitness lifestyle, you're committing to consistency and balance. So what does it take to have a sustainable relationship with health and fitness? For me, it's about having realistic and sensible goals, ones that you can maintain for years. It's the complete opposite of yo-yo diet.

This type of plan means everything is on the cards, from fruit to red meat, even cheat meals and rewards. I typically follow this type of plan after a bodybuilding competition, as it's more relaxed and it allows me to simply enjoy life and a more varied diet. **But best of all, the Balance plan is realistic. You can still drop body fat and keep your energy levels high while enjoying a sneaky treat.**

By now you're probably wondering how you can follow the Balance plan. It should be open to change, but it's important to still have some sort of a structure so that you are getting results and can stay focused. Based on my own experience, my advice is to go for an 80/20 approach. For example, for every 10 meals you eat, eight will be healthy and nutritious, including loads of vegetables, fruit, healthy carbohydrates, lean protein and fibre, but the other two will be more relaxed, like enjoying a burger or some pizza. But this doesn't mean you can pig out! Besides, at this point you hopefully don't have the urge to binge on sugar and junk food anyway, and ditching those

cravings is the main goal of following a balanced, healthy plan. The 80/20 approach also doesn't mean you get a full day off from healthy food, because that's just counterproductive. Spread your cheats out during the week.

Most importantly, make your healthy food delicious so that you'll enjoy the food you eat every single day. I adore healthy food. Give me a well-made salad loaded with homemade guacamole, shredded chicken, cashews and seeds any day. When I'm thirsty I whip up a bright and yummy juice with apple, mint, lemon and spinach. And if I want something sweet or naughty, I'll have it because it's all about balance – that's how you make this work in the long term to maintain a great body and happy mind.

The Balance plan is an enjoyable approach to healthy eating and it should be fairly effortless. Even when I'm taking a more relaxed approach, I still like to sit down on a Sunday and think about what's coming up in my week ahead, including work, meeting my friends and getting to the gym. I usually try to shop on a Sunday too so that my fridge is full of healthy and colourful foods, including things like dates, loads of fruit, Greek yoghurt, low-calorie jelly pots, wholegrain or spelt bread along with my usual suspects like rice, vegetables and protein. The one thing I don't do is buy junk food. If I'm planning on having a cheat meal, I will buy the goodies that day or go out for dinner. Having unhealthy junk food lying around will only encourage you to eat it.

Here are some tips that will help you maintain a healthy, balanced diet:

- Even if you're following this more relaxed plan, you still want to take in enough protein. A good approach that I try to follow is 1 gram of protein for every 1 kg of body weight.

- Eat five or six portions of fruit and vegetables a day, but always more vegetables than fruit.

- Drink loads of water.

- Take multivitamins and multiminerals (see page 67 for more information about these two supplements).

- Enjoy healthy carbohydrates like brown bread, brown rice, wholegrain pasta, spelt, quinoa, couscous, baby potatoes, baked potatoes and sweet potatoes.

- Keep your nutrient levels high and your brain engaged by being creative about your food and switching things up all the time. Change your breakfast around, try new recipes and try foods you have never eaten before.

- Remember the 80/20 rule: if you eat 42 meals in a week, you can have roughly eight relaxed meals or snacks. I try to only have two genuine cheat meals a week because I want to maintain my body and still look good. For my other more relaxed meals I tend to make a healthy treat like protein cookies or sweet potato brownies, protein balls or homemade granola.

- A good trick when eating cheat meals is to eat them after a big workout, especially after your leg day.

- Last but not least, be responsible about your junk food intake because you still want to get results and lose body fat or maintain your existing results. You simply cannot pig out and expect to be healthy. When I follow the Balance plan myself, the most important thing I try to remember is to eat as much healthy food as I can, keeping my sugar and salt intake fairly low and controlled.

BREAKFAST

I truly believe that breakfast is the most important meal of the day. It's the one that fuels you and gets your energy levels right. When I'm following the Balance plan, I might have a slice of toasted brown bread with avocado and a poached egg for breakfast. It's a perfect meal that includes all the major food groups. Or I might have a homemade fruit smoothie with banana, pineapple, almond milk and strawberries. Other ideas include overnight protein oats, omelettes, smoked salmon and asparagus or protein pancakes.

"SLOW RESULTS ARE MAINTAINABLE RESULTS."

EARLY LUNCH

I tend to keep this pretty quick by having something like an espresso and a low-carb protein bar. I might have an apple as well or finish off my smoothie if I didn't drink it all at breakfast. You should be relatively satisfied after your solid breakfast, so this is just to keep you going.

LUNCH

I love to make my own homemade soups packed with yummy vegetables and flavour. I might even make a giant batch and freeze it, making it healthy *and* convenient. I'll usually have a big salad on the side packed with protein, nuts, seeds, lettuce and spinach, and the odd time I might treat myself with some goat's cheese or feta.

DINNER

Get adventurous here, ladies! Remember, the Balance plan is all about enjoyment and, well, balance! Make some homemade chilli, turkey burgers or a low-calorie Thai curry. Just make sure to include protein, carbs and loads of vegetables.

SNACK

I usually have an extra meal here, but for most that would be too much. I'm a big fan of making big portions and using them throughout the day or week, so for a snack I might have some soup, salad or even something lighter like apples and peanut butter, hummus and celery or maybe even a low-calorie jelly pot if I'm feeling naughty.

To sum up, this plan is a great start and includes everything you need for a balanced and healthy lifestyle, including nutritious food, fruit and rewards. This plan will help with slow and steady weight loss that you can maintain in the long term – no more yo-yo dieting or bingeing. Feel free to switch these days around and make this plan work perfectly for your lifestyle. If I was following the Balance plan, the following table is an example of what my plan would look like, including some of the foods and dishes I enjoy eating. I've included it here so that you can use it as a guideline to create your own plan.

	MON	TUE	WED	THURS	FRI	SAT	SUN
MEAL 1	Eggs and asparagus Homemade smoothie	Chicken omelette	Protein porridge, fruit and nuts	Scrambled eggs and salmon	Protein pancakes with fruit	Green juice and spinach omelette	Poached eggs and avocado
MEAL 2	Soup and a handful of nuts	Salad and homemade juice	Soup	Salad and homemade juice	Soup and a handful of nuts	Salad and fruit smoothie	Soup
MEAL 3	Beef stir-fry	Reward (remember to be careful and control your reward)	Chicken, veg and butternut squash	Protein shake	Homemade tomato meatballs with green veg and brown rice	Protein shake and nuts	Turkey chilli con carne loaded with veg and couscous
MEAL 4	Healthy homemade Thai chicken curry with loads of green veg	Turkey burgers with brown buns and lettuce	Healthy beef burrito with veg and rice	Pitta pizza with a side of broccoli or green veg of your choice	Chicken pitta loaded with veg and a side of sweet potatoes	Grilled chicken with mango and green veg	Baked salmon with baby potatoes and veg
MEAL 5	Chicken salad	Homemade soup	Protein shake and homemade flapjacks	Reward (remember to be careful and control your reward)	Smoked salmon and asparagus	Reward (remember to be careful and control your reward)	Reward (remember to be careful and control your reward)
MEAL 6	Salad	Protein shake	Salad	Soup	Salad	Soup	Salad

MUSCLE BUILDER

Let's do it, ladies – it's time to build some serious curves.

This plan is perfect for anybody following the Booty Builder or Curve Nation plans in Chapter 8. This plan includes more food and more carbohydrates because you need the fuel to support your energy requirements for your challenging weight training sessions using heavy weights when your goal is to build lean muscle. You also want to fuel muscle growth with plenty of great food throughout the day.

When you want to build some serious curves, calories are you best friend. I read a great quote once that said, 'Calories are little creatures that live in our body and help our clothes fit better.' It's so true and it perfectly explains your mission with this plan. For example, it's impossible to build a big bum if you eat a really restricted, low-calorie diet. But that doesn't mean you get to eat a full pizza! It means eating healthy food and lots of it because you want to support lean muscle growth. I advise planning ahead, like I always do. Buy some lunch boxes, get organised and sit down on a Sunday to plan your meals for the week.

Under the Muscle Builder plan, you should be aiming to eat six meals a day. This may sound like a lot, but always remember that you should only ever eat until you're satisfied, not stuffed. You can eat up until 9 or 10 o'clock, so there are plenty of hours in the day between 7am and 10pm to eat all your meals – that's around 15 hours to play with, folks, so work in your meals around your schedule and when it suits. You don't need to be a bikini bodybuilder to eat six meals a day, and by no means is this plan going to make you bulky. You'll be eating loads of *healthy* food, not empty calories. Just remember that gaining muscle isn't easy. It's a slow process, so you must be patient.

To build muscle, the first thing you want to do is to bump up your protein intake because protein is the building block for muscle growth and it supports the repair of tissue. I typically increase my protein by an additional 0.2g to 0.5g, which means I'll try to take in a total of 1.2g or 1.5g per gram of body weight. For example, I currently weigh 62kg, so that means I'll eat roughly 74g to 93g of protein a day. It sounds like a lot, but one protein shake has 25g of protein and a chicken breast has roughly 38g. A good thing about this plan is that you can be pretty open about your sources of protein, so be adventurous and try cottage cheese, salmon, pork or duck.

Secondly, you need lots of carbs. Don't be afraid of healthy carbs like brown rice, brown pasta, sweet potatoes, oats and even some brown breads. Carbohydrates are essential for growth and energy, so eat up! I typically try to eat 3g or 4g of carbohydrates per gram of body weight, which means I eat roughly 300g of carbs a day when I want to build muscle.

And last but not least, don't forget to drink at least 2 litres of water a day and eat regular fats like fish, nuts and avocados. Using the right supplements can also help you make the most of your potential, so why not try including BCAAa, intra-workout, a protein shake post-workout and a serving of glutamine and creatine? These are some of the supplements I take during a growth period.

BREAKFAST

Always start your morning with a big breakfast that includes protein and carbs. I usually enjoy eggs with a side of spinach or asparagus along with a bowl of protein porridge. I might even shake things up a little and make a breakfast burrito with a wholegrain wrap filled with cottage cheese, scrambled eggs, sliced peppers and even turkey sausages. It's so good!

LUNCH

I tend to keep most of my meals pretty simple, so a great option for lunch is always a salad. Try a beef or chicken salad with spinach, roasted sweet potatoes and seeds.

MIDDAY MEAL

Eat something energising midday to get you through the afternoon slump. I'm a big fan of wholegrain pittas loaded with vegetable goodness, hummus and your protein of choice. Get creative – eating clean can be so enjoyable if you are prepared and organised.

DINNER

This is an important meal for me because it's typically the one I have before my workout (I like to leave about 2 hours between eating food and exercising). This particular meal is going to fuel your workout, so have something suitable, like a stir-fry with brown rice, veg and of course your protein of choice.

POST-WORKOUT MEAL

It's important to get your nutrition right just after an intense workout because it will aid recovery, which in turn supports muscle growth. Some people will have a protein shake immediately after a workout, which is a great option, but a protein shake is never a replacement for real food. I advise having a super-healthy meal post-workout, like homemade turkey meatballs and veg, or even finish off your leftovers from your pre-workout meal. Keep things convenient.

LATE MEAL

Most people don't like to eat late in the evening, and if you don't either, that's absolutely fine. Keep it light, like a bowl of chicken soup loaded with veg, which is easy to digest and not too heavy. Again, you can make all these things on a Sunday and have them ready to go in the fridge. Or you could have a casein shake right before bed. Remember, you're trying to grow muscle, so you have to consider them when you're sleeping. Casein supplies your muscles with a slow and steady release of aminos while you sleep.

Here is an example of how I would lay out the Muscle Builder plan, but again, this is just a rough guideline – use it as a springboard for creating your own plan. And remember that while this plan may seem like a lot of food, you should only eat just until you are satisfied, never to capacity. Think smaller, more functional meals and more often.

	MON	TUE	WED	THURS	FRI	SAT	SUN
MEAL 1	Eggs, asparagus and porridge	Chicken omelette and porridge	Protein porridge with pineapple and blueberries	Scrambled eggs and salmon	Protein pancakes with blueberries	Chicken breakfast burrito in a brown wrap	Poached eggs and avocado
MEAL 2	Grilled chicken with sweet potato and roasted veg	Moroccan beef burger with no bun, couscous and veg	Tuna steak with steamed veg	Salmon, brown rice and veg	White fish, greens and sweet potatoes	Garlic scrambled eggs with avocado	Turkey meatballs with brown pasta
MEAL 3	Beef stir-fry	Salad	Chicken, veg and butternut squash	Protein shake	Homemade tomato meatballs with green veg and brown rice	Protein shake and nuts	Turkey chilli con carne loaded with veg and couscous
MEAL 4	Healthy homemade Thai chicken curry with loads of green veg	Turkey burgers with brown buns and lettuce	Healthy beef burrito with veg and rice	Pitta pizza with a side of broccoli or green veg of your choice	Chicken pitta loaded with veg and a side of sweet potatoes	Grilled chicken with mango and green veg	Baked salmon with baby potatoes and veg
MEAL 5	Chicken salad	Tuna with cottage cheese and spinach	Chicken stir-fry	Cheat meal	Smoked salmon and asparagus	Cheat meal	Beef stir-fry
MEAL 6	Homemade salad	Homemade soup	Homemade soup	Homemade soup	Homemade soup	Homemade soup	Homemade soup
MEAL 7	Casein shake 35–60 minutes before bed	Casein shake 35–60 minutes before bed	Casein shake 35–60 minutes before bed	Casein shake 35–60 minutes before bed	Casein shake 35–60 minutes before bed	Casein shake 35–60 minutes before bed	Casein shake 35–60 minutes before bed

HEALTHY MIND

Eat your way to a healthy and happy mind

Just as exercise boosts your mood, food can give you a lift and increase your energy. Technically, this isn't a diet plan – it's just a guideline that encourages you to eat super-healthy foods such as fatty fish and fruits packed full of antioxidants that have been proven to assist mental health. Drink plenty of water, make sure you're taking all your vitamins and avoid stimulants like caffeine and processed foods. **Keep it natural, keep it fresh and keep it colourful.**

BREAKFAST

Start your day with a smile and a plate full of colourful, appetising food. I recommend eating some oily fish like salmon or mackerel, making a big omelette and filling it with your favourite veggies or trying a bright and colourful smoothie with strawberries, banana and goji berries.

LUNCH

Have a crunchy wholegrain wrap with lettuce, bright peppers, tomatoes, duck and homemade pesto.

AFTERNOON SNACK

In my opinion, there is nothing nicer than a big fruit bowl (I'm a fan of mango in particular). Top it with pecans, chia seeds and a big dollop of coconut yogurt. If you haven't tried coconut yogurt yet, you've been missing out!

DINNER

Steam some fish as a dinner option. As we know by now, fish is brain food, so fill up. I really like Mediterranean-style fish with vegetables and some baby potatoes with mint.

EVENING SNACK

Why not have some fun cooking up a storm in the kitchen? It always brings a smile to my face. Try making healthy falafel with hummus and veggies on the side. Or one of my favourite quick and easy snacks is apples and peanut butter.

	MON	TUE	WED	THURS	FRI	SAT	SUN
MEAL 1	Porridge with fruit and nuts	Fruit smoothie with yogurt	Greek yogurt with pineapple, nuts and flaxseeds	Garlic scrambled eggs with asparagus and smoked salmon	Greek yogurt with pineapple, nuts and flaxseeds	Porridge with fruit and nuts	Chicken and spinach omelette
MEAL 2	Wholegrain chicken pitta loaded with veg, hummus and peppers	Homemade veg soup with wholegrain bread	Herbal tea and Moroccan spiced chicken with dried fruit couscous	Wholegrain wrap with peppers and lean turkey and a side salad	Homemade flapjacks	Baked eggs and avocado	Blueberries and nuts
MEAL 3	Blueberries and nuts	Tuna with cottage cheese, peppers and spinach	Peanut butter flapjacks with blueberries	Fruit and nuts	Quinoa salad with beans and chicken	Raw veg salad with strawberries	Salmon with steamed veg and sweet potatoes
MEAL 4	Salmon with brown rice and steamed veg	Grilled chicken with mango salsa and butternut squash	Wholegrain wrap with peppers and lean turkey and a side salad	Avocado and baked eggs	Sardines with cottage cheese and spinach	Fruit and nuts	Wholegrain wrap with peppers and lean turkey and a side salad
MEAL 5	Avocado salad with tuna steak pieces and sweet potato cubes	Fruit and nuts	Steamed white fish with herbs and spices, baby potatoes and veg	Protein-packed salad	Homemade turkey burgers with wholegrain buns and salad	Lean steak and lentils	Whole wheat pasta and chicken
MEAL 6	Homemade soup with ginger and veg	Lean mince salad with spring onions	Portion of colourful fruit	Tuna steak and raw crunchy veg	Homemade soup	Apple and nut butter	Homemade soup

THE FAT BURNER

For the lady who is trying to lose a significant amount of body fat

This plan is designed for women with more experience and a good understanding of balance. It's a great one to try if you have worked with the Balance plan for at least six to 12 months and if you're looking for an extra challenge or maybe because you have a holiday coming up.

This is not a restriction diet because I don't believe in them, but you will see that there are no rewards or cheat meals mentioned (remember, these plans are not maintainable in the long term). This plan is a serious challenge, so if you are considering this one, be sure to give yourself a well-deserved but controlled reward after a long period of fat loss, then jump straight back into the Balance plan. Maximise your results by drinking as much water as possible, and try drinking herbal teas and consuming natural diuretics too – I like to eat a lot of asparagus or drink dandelion tea. One thing I really want to emphasise is that your calorie intake should still be quite high, but all of the food you'll be eating is super-healthy and lean. Low-calorie diets wreak havoc on your metabolism and you'll only end up gaining more body fat in the long term.

As I mentioned before, **losing weight is simple: just eat fewer calories than you burn**. And it doesn't need to be a painful, torturous experience. Don't forget that your body needs calories just to function, and you also want to fuel exercise. So don't even think about trying to reduce your calories as much as possible, because guess what? It's not necessary. I highly recommend checking out a calorie counter to determine a healthy

and manageable level of calories to support weight loss. I really like My Fitness Pal because it determines everything from height to exercise levels.

There are so many clever ways you can trick your body into losing body fat without making drastic changes. Try carb cycling (see page 166–167), switching your regular milk to almond milk or even increasing your exercise by an additional 15 minutes. Every little change will help you reduce your calorie intake or burn more calories.

Here is an example of how I would plan my diet day if I was being super good. And remember, these types of plans are only meant to be followed for the short term, such as four weeks. Then you can jump straight back to the Balance plan, which is important if you want to maintain your fitness in the long term.

BREAKFAST

When I'm trying to shift some extra body fat, I like to manipulate my carbohydrate intake. Carbs are important – you need them for energy. I typically eat carbs around the middle of the day, so in the morning I'll have a giant mug of mint, dandelion or nettle tea. These are cleansing and natural diuretics, which will help reduce bloating. For breakfast, I'll usually eat an omelette made with one egg yolk and three egg whites with a side of steamed asparagus. Just because you're eating clean doesn't mean your food should be bland, so throw in all kinds of herbs and colourful vegetables – the more veg you eat, the better! Other things I like to eat in the morning are turkey sausages, turkey bacon, avocados and roasted veg. I might also have a protein isolate shake for a fast-absorbing protein source to start my day.

MIDDAY MEALS

I like to eat regularly throughout the day when I follow a plan like this because it really helps to stop any potential cravings for junk food and it keeps your blood sugar levels stable. I'll eat a range of meals during the day, but because I'm being extra good under this plan, I like to eat green vegetables, a lean protein source and healthy carbohydrates. I tend to avoid red meat when I'm following this plan, as your body digests it more slowly, so I'll stick with turkey or chicken and switch my carb source from brown breads and white potatoes to sweet potatoes or quinoa. An example of a meal that I might eat when I'm following this plan is shepherd's pie made with minced turkey breast and mashed sweet potatoes and loaded with greens, or a Mexican rice and chicken salad.

Again, there's no reason to eat bland food, no matter what diet plan you're following. There are so many books and sources online with recipes for all sorts of healthy food, from salads to chilli or even burgers. If food tastes bad, you won't stick to your diet plan, plain and simple. One tip is to be organised – bring lunch boxes to work or go to a healthy café for lunch. Just be ready so that you have no excuses to make bad food choices.

You'll also notice that because your meals including carbohydrates are in the middle of the day, you should do your exercise during this time too, as you'll need those carbs for energy. You will also see some carb cycling thrown in to help you shed some extra body fat. Remember, low-carb days are for resting, so make sure your workout plan matches.

EVENING MEALS

I really like using carb cycling. There are so many different ways you can do it, but reducing your carb intake in the evenings is a pretty easy way to approach it. If I'm eating six or seven meals a day, I'll reduce my carbs in my last meal or two by eating a chicken salad with peppers, cucumber and a load of other bright vegetables, or I might have a homemade mint pea soup.

A good supplements plan with a multivitamin and multimineral tablet is an important part of this diet plan too. Why not try one thermogenic fat burner with breakfast during these four weeks as a little boost on top of your workout and diet plan?

Here are some final tips:

- Eat often.

- Eat loads of greens.

- Drink as much water as possible.

- Be organised.

- Manipulate your carb intake, but never cut them out altogether.

- Swap red meat for fish, chicken or turkey.

- Don't restrict your diet. Keep your calories high enough to support your daily requirements, but keep your food healthy.

- Reduce cheat meals and rewards – try having only one a week if you really need it.

- This sort of approach is for the short term only. Try it for four weeks, then go back to the Balance plan.

- Try increasing your exercise. For example, on top of your gym workout, throw in a 20- or 30-minute walk with your girlfriends or your dog.

The following table is a very basic guideline that gives you the freedom to pick your favourite protein sources, greens and carbs. As you can see, it uses carb cycling, so there are fewer carbs in the evening and in the morning. When following this fat-burning plan, you just have to eat six meals a day and include every food group. Simple!

	MON	TUE	WED	THURS	FRI	SAT	SUN
MEAL 1	Protein isolate shake with eggs and green veg	Protein isolate shake with eggs and green veg	Protein isolate shake with eggs and green veg	Protein isolate shake with eggs and green veg	Protein isolate shake with eggs and green veg	Protein isolate shake with eggs and green veg	Protein isolate shake with eggs and green veg
MEAL 2	Protein with green veg and carbs	Protein with green veg and carbs	Protein with green veg and carbs	Protein with green veg and carbs	Protein with green veg and carbs	Protein with green veg and carbs	Protein with green veg and carbs
MEAL 3	Protein with green veg, carbs and fats	Protein with green veg and carbs	Protein with green veg, carbs and fats	Protein with green veg and carbs	Protein with green veg and carbs	Protein with green veg and fats	Protein with green veg, carbs and fats
MEAL 4	Protein with green veg and carbs	Protein with green veg and carbs	Protein with green veg and carbs	Protein with green veg and carbs	Protein with green veg	Protein with green veg and fats	Protein with green veg and carbs
MEAL 5	Protein with green veg and carbs	Protein with green veg	Protein with green veg	Protein with green veg	Protein with green veg	Protein with green veg and fats	Protein with green veg
MEAL 6	Protein with green veg	Protein with green veg	Protein with green veg	Protein with green veg	Protein with green veg	Protein with green veg	Protein with green veg

FUNCTIONAL EATING

Functional eating is way of maximising results by interlinking food and exercise, and making the most out of both using clever techniques. It's not essential, but it can be a big help if you want to get the most out of your efforts. This is for people who have really got to grips with a healthy lifestyle and are ready to take it to the next level.

Think of functional eating as eating like an athlete. According to books like *Food, Nutrition and Sports Performance III* by R.J. Maughan and S. M. Shirreffs and *The Functional Foods Revolution: Healthy People, Healthy Profits* by J. Mellentin and M. Heasman, the theory is that your metabolism is not fixed throughout the day, so you should eat accordingly. It's also about using fuel to maximise your workout results.

To eat functionally:

- Always eat a breakfast that includes protein.

- Eat more carbohydrates between waking up and 2pm.

- Reduce carbohydrates in the evening and increase your protein portion to replace them.

Your pre-workout fuel is the last meal you have before your workout, so it will be the main source of energy for your workout. This is important, as you want to be sharp and focused and to make the most of your training. By eating a meal with both carbs and protein in it, you will stop muscle protein breakdown and optimise glycogen levels, which gives you the energy to train. Ideally, you should consume food 1–1.5 hours before your workout.

Intra-workout fuel is focused on sustenance during your workout with the goal of supporting the muscles. The most convenient intra-workout option is branch chain amino acids (BCAAs). Having an intra-workout shake can support muscle growth and recovery, help avoid delayed onset muscle soreness and also increase stamina and performance during a workout.

Post-workout fuel is the golden hour that you'd better take advantage of if you want functional eating to help you improve your results. As the name suggests, post-workout fuel takes place immediately after a workout, when you can exploit the anabolic state your body is in. The main goal of this period is to replenish the glycogen lost during the workout along with muscle recovery and repair. The most effective post-workout product is a whey protein shake because it's quickly absorbed, which means protein gets to your muscles more quickly. Have one whey protein shake no later than 20 to 30 minutes after your workout. You can also add one serving of glutamine and one serving of creatine on top of that if you are really looking to build some sexy muscle (more on those in the next chapter).

CARB CYCLING AND CARB MANIPULATION

This technique is for the woman who has mastered eating a healthy and balanced diet plan for at least one year. Once you have mastered the basics, then you can take the next step and use carb cycling as an extra tool in your arsenal to help you torch body fat. As you know, the way to burn body fat is to burn more calories than you consume, but this is a clever little tool that can really help you in the next level of your journey. The idea is to manipulate your carbohydrate consumption around your training, a technique that supports muscle growth along with maximum fat loss without restricting yourself.

High-carb day: This is the day with the highest amount of carbohydrates, so it's also the perfect day for cheat meals if you decide to take this approach because it's the day you will have the most challenging workouts, which are usually legs. Your carbohydrate intake could be anywhere up to 200g or more a day (typically 2g per pound of body weight).

Moderate carb days: As your carbohydrates decrease, both your protein and fat intake should increase. There should always be a balance (look at the pie chart on page 148 again) and you should never be restricted in terms of calories for the day. Your moderate day will be to fuel exercise and normal function, but will have a slight decrease in comparison to a high-carb day. Your moderate day could be 150g–180g using 1.5g per pound of body weight.

Low-carb days: Low-carb days are the days when you take in the least amount of carbohydrates, but again, it's not an excuse to restrict or starve yourself. Your protein and fat intake will have increased significantly to support normal function and to replace the reduced amount of carbs. Low-carb days work best during rest days because you need fewer carbs since you aren't doing as much activity. Low-carb days should be immediately followed with high-carb days to replenish body function and hormone balance. A low-carb day could be 60–100g of protein, based on 0.5g per pound of body weight.

The grams guidelines above are totally changeable and are a personal thing. If you're trying this technique, keep a diary of how you feel on the three different days. It may take a couple of goes to find out how your body reacts best, but here are two examples of how you could plan it.

OPTION 1

MONDAY	Lower body workout	High carbs
TUESDAY	Upper body workout	Moderate carbs
WEDNESDAY	Rest day	Low carbs
THURSDAY	Upper body workout	Moderate carbs
FRIDAY	Lower body workout	High carbs
SATURDAY	Cardio day	Moderate carbs
SUNDAY	Rest day	Low carbs

OPTION 2

MONDAY	Leg day	High carbs
TUESDAY	Back day	High carbs
WEDNESDAY	Triceps and biceps	Moderate carbs
THURSDAY	Glutes and abs	Moderate carbs
FRIDAY	Shoulders and chest	Moderate carbs
SATURDAY	Rest day	Moderate carbs
SUNDAY	Rest day	Low carbs

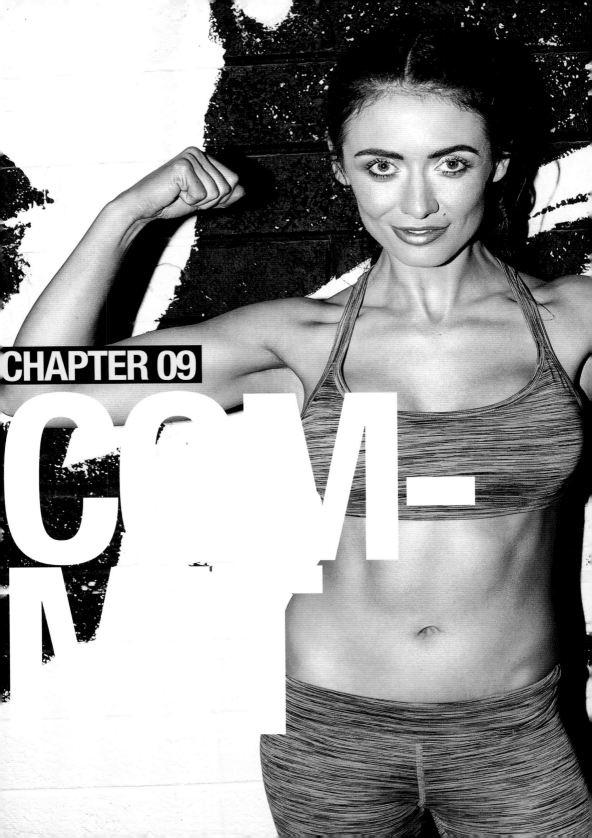

CHAPTER 09

COM-
M

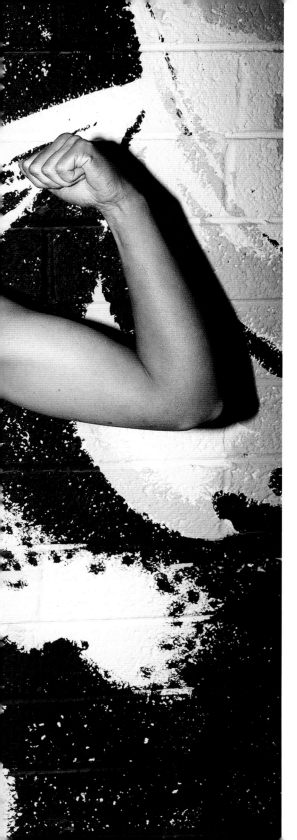

Writing down your goals, dreams and even your insecurities is a proactive way to start your fitness journey and figure out how to effect change. I want *BYOB* to be more than just a book – I want it to be an interactive guide that will help you improve, but you can't make improvements if you don't know exactly what your goals are. This chapter gives you a chance to think about them. It might take you a while to answer all the questions, but give it a go. By the time you've filled out each section, you will feel 100% ready to take on your new fitness endeavours.

Be kind to yourself, be honest, be ready to work and be prepared to push yourself. You need to be able to give yourself constructive criticism too – don't go easy on yourself! And don't tolerate mediocrity, because with the right attitude, you can be the best version of yourself. All of these things will help you identify how to improve and boost your confidence.

Use this section as a personal fitness diary and a tool to give you clarity in a fun and self-loving way. It's something you can write in when you feel inspired and also something you can look back on for motivation. You are already incredible, so write it down. **Self-confidence starts in your own mind and heart.** Answer the questions and put your thoughts down on paper, because sometimes you have to put those words out into the universe to make them happen.

20 REASONS WHY YOU ARE AMAZING

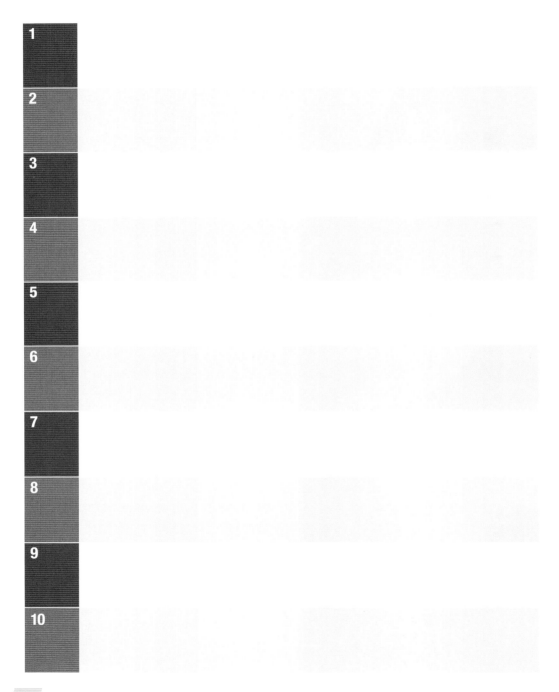

1

2

3

4

5

6

7

8

9

10

11

12

13

14

15

16

17

18

19

20

10 WEAKNESSES THAT YOU CAN IMPROVE ON

1

2

3

4

5

6

7

8

9

10

10 EXCUSES YOU HAVE USED IN THE PAST THAT YOU WON'T USE NOW OR IN THE FUTURE

1

2

3

4

5

6

7

8

9

10

10 REASONS YOU ARE GOING TO SUCCEED NOW AND IN THE FUTURE

1

2

3

4

5

6

7

8

9

10

YOUR SHORT-TERM HEALTH AND FITNESS GOALS

1

2

3

4

5

6

7

8

9

10

YOUR LONG-TERM HEALTH AND FITNESS GOALS

1

2

3

4

5

6

7

8

9

10

WHAT IS YOUR BIGGEST GOAL(S) FOR THIS YEAR?

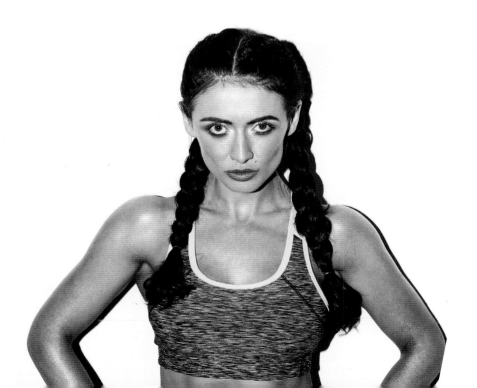

FIVE WAYS YOU ARE GOING TO MAKE YOUR GOALS HAPPEN

1

2

3

4

5

WHAT IS YOUR GOAL FOR NEXT YEAR?

WHAT IS YOUR GOAL FOR THE YEAR AFTER THAT?

DO YOU HAVE ANY MEDICAL CONDITIONS OR INJURIES THAT MIGHT NEED TO BE ADDRESSED BEFORE STARTING?

WRITE A MESSAGE TO YOURSELF FOR TIMES WHEN YOU ARE UNMOTIVATED

WRITE A MESSAGE TO YOUR PAST SELF

HOW CAN YOU FURTHER IMPROVE YOUR HEALTH AND FITNESS KNOWLEDGE?

TICK THE FOODS YOU LOVE, LIKE OR ARE GOING TO TRY

VEGETABLES	FRUIT	MEAT, FISH AND EGGS	CARBOHY-DRATES	NUTS, OILS AND SEEDS
☐ Artichoke	☐ Apple	☐ Chicken breast	☐ Brown bread	☐ Almond butter
☐ Asparagus	☐ Banana	☐ Eggs	☐ Brown pasta	☐ Almonds
☐ Aubergine	☐ Blueberries	☐ Lean steak	☐ Brown rice	☐ Cashew butter
☐ Avocado	☐ Grapefruit	☐ Prawns	☐ Butter beans	☐ Cashews
☐ Broccoli	☐ Grapes	☐ Salmon	☐ Chickpeas	☐ Chia seeds
☐ Brussels sprouts	☐ Kiwi	☐ Squid	☐ Couscous	☐ Coconut oil
☐ Cabbage	☐ Lemon	☐ Tinned tuna	☐ Lentils	☐ Flaxseeds
☐ Carrot	☐ Lime	☐ Tuna steak	☐ Oats	☐ Hazelnuts
☐ Cauliflower	☐ Mango	☐ Turkey	☐ Sweet potatoes	☐ Olive oil
☐ Celery	☐ Melon	☐ White fish	☐ White potatoes	☐ Peanut butter
☐ Courgette	☐ Orange		☐ White rice	☐ Peanuts
☐ Green beans	☐ Peach			☐ Pecans
☐ Kale	☐ Pear			☐ Pistachios
☐ Lettuce	☐ Pineapple			☐ Walnuts
☐ Mushrooms	☐ Raspberries			
☐ Peas	☐ Strawberries			
☐ Peppers				
☐ Rocket				
☐ Spinach				
☐ Tomatoes				
☐ Turnip				

LIST YOUR TRIGGERS (WE ALL HAVE THEM!)

1

2

3

4

5

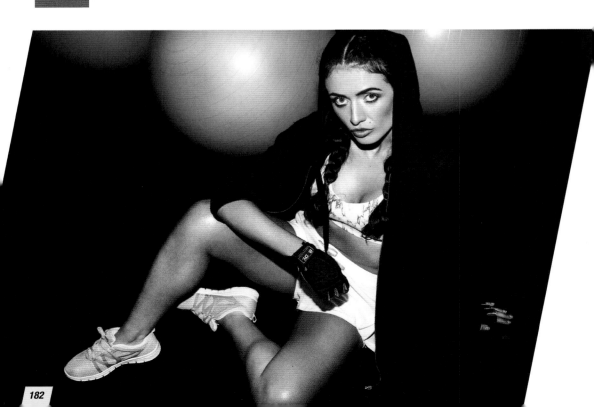

WHAT IS YOUR WEEKLY SCHEDULE LIKE?

MONDAY

TUESDAY

WEDNESDAY

THURSDAY

FRIDAY

SATURDAY

SUNDAY

WHAT DAYS SUIT YOU BEST TO EXERCISE?

MONDAY	Morning	Midday	Afternoon
TUESDAY	Morning	Midday	Afternoon
WEDNESDAY	Morning	Midday	Afternoon
THURSDAY	Morning	Midday	Afternoon
FRIDAY	Morning	Midday	Afternoon
SATURDAY	Morning	Midday	Afternoon
SUNDAY	Morning	Midday	Afternoon

WHAT DAY WILL YOU DO YOUR HEALTHY SHOP AND THINK ABOUT YOUR FOOD FOR THE WEEK?

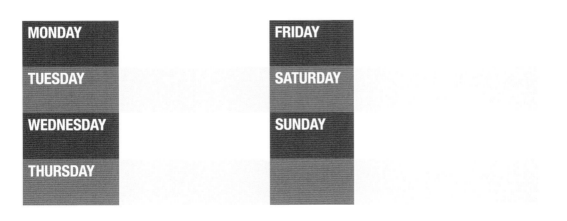

MONDAY	FRIDAY
TUESDAY	SATURDAY
WEDNESDAY	SUNDAY
THURSDAY	

WHAT CAN YOU PLAN OR SIGN UP FOR THAT WILL KEEP YOU MOTIVATED?

WHICH *BYOB* WORKOUT PLAN ARE YOU GOING TO FOLLOW AND FOR HOW LONG?

WHICH *BYOB* DIET PLAN WILL YOU FOLLOW AND FOR HOW LONG?

WHAT WILL YOUR FOLLOW-UP DIET PLAN BE?

WHICH OF THE FOLLOWING MOST APPLIES TO YOU?

A social butterfly who depends on the energy of others

Class exercise or sports

An independent girl who doesn't need anybody except herself

Solo workout gal

You hate classes but need support

A workout buddy is essential

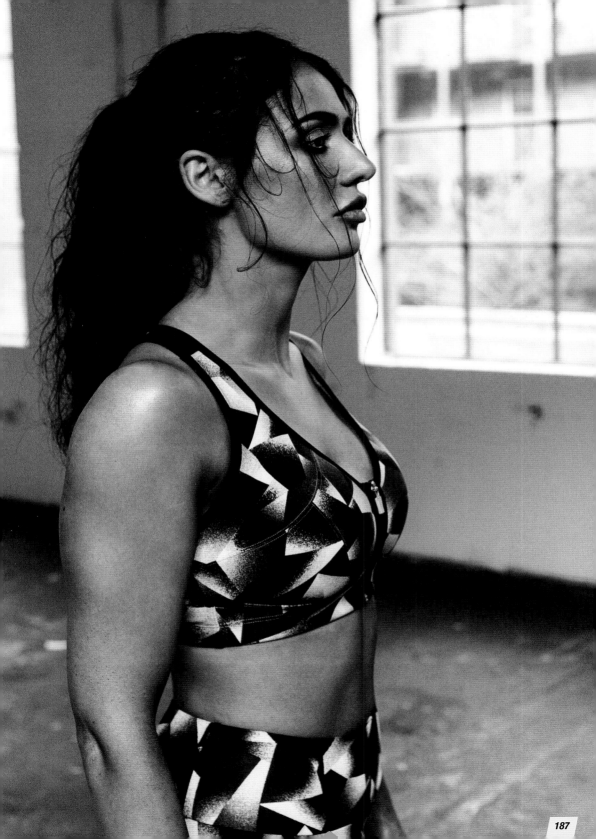

DESIGN YOUR *BYOB* WORKOUT PLAN

PLAN 1

MON	TUES	WED	THURS	FRI	SAT	SUN

PLAN 2

MON	TUES	WED	THURS	FRI	SAT	SUN

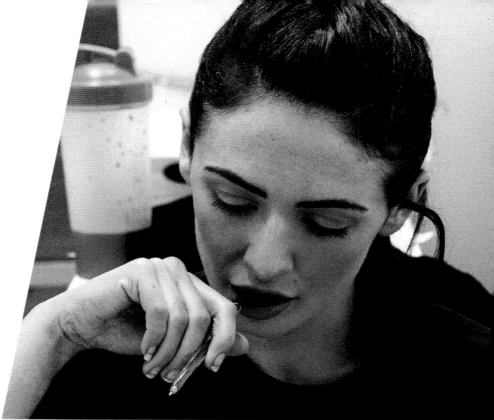

DESIGN YOUR *BYOB* DIET PLAN BASED ON YOUR CALORIE NEEDS

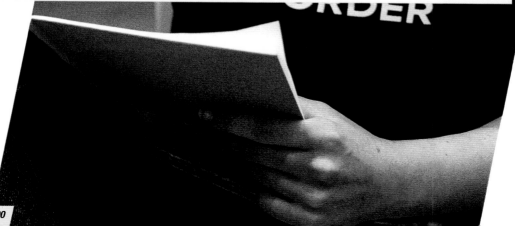

What are your calorie needs for the day?

How many grams of protein do you need a day?

How many grams of carbohydrates do you need a day?

How many grams of fats do you need a day?

PLAN 1

MON	TUES	WED	THURS	FRI	SAT	SUN

PLAN 2

MON	TUES	WED	THURS	FRI	SAT	SUN

WHAT SUPPLEMENTS DO YOU PLAN ON TAKING?

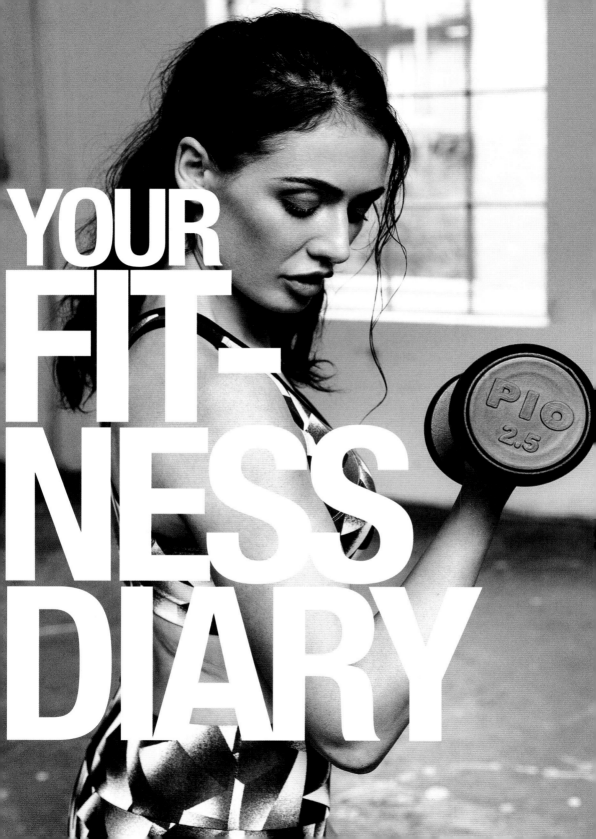

FURTHER READING

COOKBOOKS AND BOOKS ABOUT FOOD

Deliciously Ella: Awesome Ingredients, Incredible Food That You and Your Body Will Love
by Ella Woodward

Everyday Super Food
by Jamie Oliver

In Defense of Food: An Eater's Manifesto
by Michael Pollan

It's All Good: Delicious, Easy Recipes That Will Make You Look Good and Feel Great
by Gwyneth Paltrow

The Body Fat Solution: Five Principles for Burning Fat, Building Lean Muscle, Ending Emotional Eating, and Maintaining Your Perfect Weight
by Tom Venuto

The Chopra Center Cookbook: Nourishing Body and Soul
by Deepak Chopra

The Fit Bottomed Girl's Anti-Diet
by Jennipher Walters

The Honest Life: Living Naturally and True to You
by Jessica Alba

The Master Your Metabolism Cookbook
by Jillian Michaels

The Shredded Chef: 120 Recipes for Building Muscle, Getting Lean, and Staying Health
by Michael Matthews

EXERCISE, WEIGHT LOSS AND MUSCLE-BUILDING BOOKS

Bigger Leaner Stronger: The Simple Science of Building the Ultimate Male Body
by Michael Matthews

Hardcore Bodybuilding: A Scientific Approach
by Frederick Hatfield

Journal of Strength and Conditioning Research

Making the Cut: The 30-Day Diet and Fitness Plan for the Strongest, Sexiest You
by Jillian Michaels

Sculpting Her Body Perfect
by Brad Schoenfeld

Slim for Life: My Insider Secrets to Simple, Fast, and Lasting Weight Loss
by Jillian Michaels

Strength Training Anatomy
by Frederic Delavier

The New Encyclopedia of Modern Bodybuilding: The Bible of Bodybuilding
by Arnold Schwarzenegger

Thinner Leaner Stronger: The Simple Science of Building the Ultimate Female Body
by Michael Matthews

OTHER BOOKS WORTH CHECKING OUT

#GIRLBOSS
by Sophia Amoruso

My Fight/Your Fight
by Ronda Rousey

The Marshmallow Test: Why Self-Control Is the Engine of Success
by Walter Mischel

Wild: From Lost to Found on the Pacific Crest Trail
by Cheryl Strayed

PODCASTS

The Jillian Michaels Show
The Mike Dolce Show

WEBSITES

Bodybuilding.com
Fitnessgurls.com
Muscleandfitness.com
Shape.com
Tnation.com
Womenshealth.com
Womenshealthmag.co.uk

Leabharlanna Poibli Chathair Bhaile Átha Cliath
Dublin City Public Libraries